Victor Moebus Farias
Luiz Antonio Moura Keller
Robson Maia Franco

EVALUATION OF THE QUALITY OF INFANT FORMULAS OFFERED TO NEONATES

Victor Moebus Farias
Luiz Antonio Moura Keller
Robson Maia Franco

EVALUATION OF THE QUALITY OF INFANT FORMULAS OFFERED TO NEONATES

Microbiological and toxicological analysis

ScienciaScripts

Imprint

Any brand names and product names mentioned in this book are subject to trademark, brand or patent protection and are trademarks or registered trademarks of their respective holders. The use of brand names, product names, common names, trade names, product descriptions etc. even without a particular marking in this work is in no way to be construed to mean that such names may be regarded as unrestricted in respect of trademark and brand protection legislation and could thus be used by anyone.

Cover image: www.ingimage.com

This book is a translation from the original published under ISBN 978-620-5-50281-5.

Publisher:
Sciencia Scripts
is a trademark of
Dodo Books Indian Ocean Ltd. and OmniScriptum S.R.L Publishing group
Str. Armeneasca 28/1, office 1, Chisinau MD-2012, Republic of Moldova, Europe
Printed at: see last page
ISBN: 978-620-5-38514-2

THANKS

To the Universidade Federal Fluminense, the laboratory of Microbiological Control of Products of Animal Origin (LCMPOA), the department of Food Technology - MTA of the Veterinary School of UFP.

To the Graduate Program in Veterinary Medicine at UFF, for the support during the development of the research.

To the Coordination for the Improvement of Higher Education Personnel (CAPES) for the scholarship granted for the studies.

To my supervisor, Robson Maia Franco, for the knowledge passed, for the advice, for the long conversations and laughs, for the affection and for accepting me as a student in the course.

To my advisor, Luiz Antonio Moura Keller, for opening these doors for me, for the support and encouragement, for always being present and being more than an advisor.

To the Chief of the Nutrition Service of the Antônio Pedro University Hospital for access to the lactation unit and for providing the samples, and to the technicians and servers of the sector for preparing the samples.

To Drs. Eliane Rodrigues and Marcos Aronovich, and the laboratory of the State Center for Research in Food Quality (CEPQA) / PESAGRO - Rio, for the possibility of training since graduation and the use of space for this project

To Professor Kelly Keller, and the Laboratory of Mycology and Mycotoxins (LAMICO) at the Federal University of Minas Gerais, for conducting the toxicological analyses of this project.

To Professor Eliana Mesquita, for the support, encouragement, ear pulling; for the conversations and jokes.

To my family, for always waiting for me and welcoming me on weekends, with delicious food in the oven and fresh coffee.

To my dear Camilla, for all her love and companionship and support. For being the best girlfriend in the world, for the patience and encouragement in completing this project, and for always being by my side supporting me in new projects.

To my brother Matheus, for his support, company, late night chats and for being the best copilot one could ever want

To my undergraduate friends, for being with me at every moment throughout all these years.

To my friends, Beatriz Clarissa and Leonardo Pinto, for their help in several parts of the project.

To all X-family, for being more than friends in Niterói.

To my friends from Lan & House, for all the support and understanding for the missed meetings.

To the whole CEPQA team, for all the support, encouragement, advice and technical and academic teachings in all these years.

To the colleagues from the Fish Laboratory and the Animal Health and Toxicology Centre for all their companionship.

To the post-graduation companions, for the conviviality and companionship during the disciplines.

To the boys of the Reach for forming a family in Niterói.

SUMMARY

Due to the changes suffered by society and its rhythm, eating habits are being altered and increasingly neglected, especially infant feeding. If becoming necessary the inclusion of infant formulas in the diet of children, especially newborns. Considering the fragility of the target population, it is important to carry out studies for the evaluation of possible microbiological and toxicological hazards to which consumers are exposed as well as the relevance of such hazards. The microbiological and toxicological quality of infant formulas for early childhood, offered by the lactation unit of the Antônio Pedro University Hospital, Fluminense Federal University, were evaluated. The counts of mesophilic aerobic heterotrophic bacteria (MBHAM), enterobacteria, lactic acid bacteria, coagualase positive *Staphylococcus, Bacillus cereus,* Most Probable Number (MPN) of total coliforms and research of *Salmonella* spp. were performed, as described in the APHA manual (2015). MPN of *Enterococcus* spp. according to Merck manual and *Cronobacter sakazakii research* according to the methodology described by the ISSO/TS 22964 standard. The research of filamentous fungi and xerophilic fungi was performed using DRBC and DG18 media, respectively, following the methodology proposed by Pitt and Hocking (1998) and Abarca (1994). The determination of aflatoxin M1 was carried out by fluorimetry after extraction associated with immuno-enzymatic methods. After the evaluation of the 36 samples, lactic acid bacteria, *B. cereus, C. sakazakii,* coliforms, enterobacteriaceae, *Enterococcus* spp. and *Salmonella spp. were* not detected in any of the samples. From the analysis revealed mean values (CFU/mL): mesophilic aerobes of 3.54×10^3 ; coagulase positive Staphylococcus 3.89×10^1 ; filamentous and xerophilic fungi 8.14×10^2 and 2.34×103, respectively. The data obtained in the study proved the safety of the food and the compliance with the current legislation, corroborating the recommendations for immediate consumption after re-suspension of the product, as well as the recommendations for storage of the product in order to avoid the proliferation of pathogenic microorganisms. The quantification of aflatoxin M1 in all analyzed samples remained below the detection limit of the technique (<0.013 mg/kg), being below the recommended by the legislation, not offering risk to the consumer. The count values obtained in this study may be interpreted as a reflection of flaws during product processing, choice of raw material and handling during reconstitution. However, in the samples analysed, the count values were found to be within the levels recommended by legislation, thus being in conformity and safe for consumption.

Key words: Infant formulas, fungal count, *Salmonella* spp., aflatoxin M1, *Cronobacter sakazakii*

SUMMARY

1 INTRODUCTION

According to the World Health Organization (WHO), the importance of exclusive breastfeeding is recommended in the first six months of life, followed by continued breastfeeding with complementary foods for up to two years or more (WHO, 2003). Breastfeeding can be classified as total if only breast milk is given, mixed if infant formulas are also given, and partial if breastfeeding is accompanied by complementary foods (GUERRA et al., 2012).

Breastfeeding is extremely important for newborns due to its nutritional potential: helping to fight infections, as well as developing the newborn's immune system (VICTORIA et al., 1987). The society as a whole has been undergoing changes and entering more and more into an accelerated rhythm. The accelerated rhythm of modern life is not conducive to the creation of healthy eating habits, as it leads to an increasing intake of processed and industrialized foods. With this, the insertion of women into the labour market, and often the need to return to work activities, ends up reducing the breastfeeding period, leading to the need for food supplementation.

According to the National Health Surveillance Agency (ANVISA) foods for enteral nutrition supplementation, are defined as those intended to supplement the diet of an individual, when necessary, and may not, however, replace the food itself (BRASIL, 2018). Like any food, food supplements can also present risks to the population. Whether in the form of biological hazards, such as the presence of bacteria and fungi. As well as residues of chemical substances, potential inducers of poisoning and allergenic processes.

Therefore, it is necessary to carry out studies on the risks in order to know and evaluate them within the safety limits for the target population. Studies that evaluate and monitor these matrices, as to risks and contaminants, attest not only to the standard of identity and quality of products, but also subsidise the community with important data when it comes to widely consumed products.

2 THEORETICAL FOUNDATION

2.1 NEWBORNS: BREAST MILK AND BREASTFEEDING

Human milk is the only food ingested in sufficient quantities by newborns that has high nutritional, energy and immunological value. Breast milk is important for the newborn's growth and development, in addition to assisting in the formation of the immune system, nervous system, and facilitating emotional and cognitive development (WHO, 2018). The first contact between mother and child has priority importance in the humanised vision of baby care in the delivery room. In order to avoid unnecessary separations, which could harm breastfeeding and the baby's closeness, it is important to reduce the procedures performed in the immediate postpartum period to what is strictly necessary, when it concerns a low-risk baby (CRUZ; SUMAN; SPÍNDOLA, 2007).

The nutritional composition of human milk has a lipid value above 3%, accounting for about 50% of the caloric value of food (VIEIRA et al., 2004). It is an excellent source of cholesterol, essential fatty acids and vitamins (INNIS; DYER; NELSON, 1994).

Due to the metabolism of the newborn child, a high protein intake is necessary, especially during the first months of life. Breast milk has a protein content of about 1.2%. About 60 to 90% of this content is serum protein, with approximately half of the concentration made up of alpha-lactalbumin, which is needed for iron transport (CALIL; FALCÃO, 2003). Human milk also contains high concentrations of essential amino acids of high biological value, such as cystine and taurine, which are important for the development of the central nervous system. This is important for premature babies, as they are unable to synthesize them due to enzyme deficiencies (SILVA; ESCOBEDO; GIOIELLI, 2007).

Due to nutritional and cognitive characteristics, maternal breastfeeding in the first months is encouraged by international bodies and the use of supplementary foods is not recommended, except in some situations. The medical reasons listed in the international recommendations as acceptable for the use of supplementary or replacement foods are exceptions: very low birth weight newborns (< 1,500g), premature infants with less than 32 weeks of gestational age, those who cannot gain weight or maintain the degree of hydration with breast milk alone, those whose mother has a serious illness or is on medication that is contraindicated during breastfeeding, and those with inborn errors of metabolism (WHO, 2009a).

2.2 INFANT FORMULAE

2.2.1 **Legislation**

Food supplements, according to ANVISA, are products for oral ingestion, presented in pharmaceutical forms, intended to supplement the diet of healthy individuals with nutrients, bioactive substances, enzymes or probiotics, alone or in combination (BRASIL, 2018). The definition was drafted based on the *Codex Alimentarius* guidelines (FAO, 2005), and international standards such as the Food and Drug Administration (FDA), which defines a food supplement as a product intended to supplement the diet that contains one or more of the following dietary ingredients: vitamin, mineral, herbal or other botanical product and amino acids (FDA, 1995). Among the age groups, there are two groups in which supplementation is more necessary, the elderly and newborns.

The formulas used in the supplementation of newborns can be defined as a product, in liquid or powder form, used when indicated, for healthy infants from the sixth month of life until twelve months of incomplete age (11 months and 29 days) and for healthy early childhood children, constituting the main liquid element of a progressively diversified diet (BRASIL, 2011a).

In the Collegiate Resolution (RDC) No. 44 of 2011, the repeal of Ordinance No. 977 of 1998 of the Ministry of Health is included due to updates of the *Codex Alimentarius* and advances in research and new discoveries on the subject. However, the new RDC does not include the microbiological quality standards and residue control in products, being the microbiological standard contained in item 25 of RDC No. 12 of 2001 (BRASIL, 2001) and the mycotoxin limits in RDC No. 07 of 2011 (BRASIL, 2011b).

The limits of drug residues are determined by two programs. The Ministry of Agriculture acts through the National Plan for the Control of Residues in Products of Animal Origin (PNCR) (BRASIL, 1999), while ANVISA acts with the National Programme of Analysis of Residues of Veterinary Drugs in Food Exposed to Consumption (PAMvet) (BRASIL, 2003a).

2.2.2 Components and potential aggregate risks

Food safety has been an imposition in the context of international trade of agricultural and livestock products, being the consumers' health the world priority, and, as a consequence, the quality of raw material used in food production. It is important to take into consideration the ingredients used in the production, such as whey protein, the main source of protein of the supplements studied and product of animal origin of higher concentration, which may be associated with various microorganisms, including bacteria of the coliform group, *Escherichia coli* and *Staphylococcus aureus* (ALIJALOUD et al., 2013; CORTEZ et al., 2013).

Components of plant origin can also be associated with fungi such as the genus *Aspergillus,* often related to the production of toxins (GERMANO; GERMANO, 2011).

The mycotoxins found may also be associated with the genera *Fusarium* and *Penicillium,* and may originate both from vegetable and animal products and, although they are not often associated with acute conditions, prolonged ingestion is related to chronic infections. All these factors are risk factors for the immunocompromised consumer and must be elucidated (DILKIN, 2002; FORSYTHE, 2002).

Another issue worth mentioning is the presence of antimicrobial residues, such as p-lactams, tetracycline and aminoglycosides. The residues make the food unfit for human consumption since they can lead to allergies, with continuous ingestion compromising the immune, endocrine and nervous systems, suppressing bone marrow and increasing the risk of cancer (AYTENFSU; MAMO; KEBEDE, 2016). The development of bacterial resistance by ingesting food containing residues can influence the patient's treatment, leading to failures and relapse, as well as the use of drugs of greater toxicity to the patient (BRODY, 2006).

In 2005, the Ministry of Health implemented in Brazil the Program of Analysis of Residues of Veterinary Drugs in Food in which listed the groups of antimicrobials that should be monitored in dairy matrices. In the report issued in 2009, it is highlighted the research of the following groups of antibiotics: p-lactams, tetracyclines, amfenicols, aminoglycosides and macrolides (BRASIL, 2009).

2.2.3 **Nutritional components of infant formulae**

According to FAO (2008), the best options for replacing breast milk are infant formulas when breastfeeding is not possible. Therefore, numerous products have been developed and formulated to meet the nutritional deficiencies resulting from the ingestion of breast milk.

Nowadays, the industry has advanced technology available to manufacture various types of infant formulas for each segment, but it is impossible to reproduce human milk. Due to the variation of nutrients in the raw materials used in the preparation of infant formulas, such as bovine milk and soybeans, it was established that infant formulas should present nutrient levels similar to those presented in breast milk (FAO, 2008; KASHLAN et al, 1991).

Infant formulas usually have bovine milk as the basic raw material. As milk is not suitable for newborn babies, the raw material needs to be subjected to technological processing to improve digestion and absorption (MOURA, 2007).

Due to the difference between the osmolarity of bovine and human milk, the milk, before thermal processing, is diluted to an osmolarity similar to human milk. Most formulas include lactose, sucrose, corn syrup (fructose) and/or maltose-dextrin and others add starch from different sources, as a way to compensate the concentration of total solids in the product (FOMON, 1987; MOURA, 2007).

After dilution, whole milk is submitted to thermal treatment to obtain the dehydrated product in order to increase its durability due to the reduction of the water activity and, consequently, its availability to participate in the chemical, biochemical and microbiological transformations (JENSEN, 2002).

When it comes to proteins, besides the initial milk dilution, it is necessary to add proteins, either whey proteins or demineralized whey. This addition aims to improve the whey protein/casein ratio of the final product, since the concentration of casein in bovine milk is twice as high as in breast milk (MAHAN et al., 1998).

The addition of taurine, present in human milk and absent in bovine milk, has been made in some formulations because of its role in brain and retinal development and formation in newborns. In infant formulas for specific dietary needs, formulations are developed with hydrolysed lacto- albumin and added amino acids. In cases of allergy to protein of animal origin, the protein base used is soy protein, which is also highly allergenic (MOURA, 2007).

The addition of vegetable oils aims to increase the concentration of essential fatty acids when using skimmed milks for the manufacture of infant formulas. Due to this addition, infant formulas have a high ratio of polyunsaturated/saturated fatty acids and little or no cholesterol (ESCOBAR et al, 2002).

During dilution, the concentration of minerals in the milk is reduced to levels close to those of mother's milk. This is necessary because of the excess of minerals in bovine milk, such as sodium, which has a concentration three times higher than in human milk, making partial demineralisation necessary as a complementary step (LONNERDAL, 2000).

The iron content in both types of milk is similar, but bovine milk does not have heme iron and, therefore, there are losses during the absorption of this mineral (COSTA; MONTEIRO, 2004). Moura (2007) observed in his study that bovine milk also has the ability to inhibit the absorption of iron, in both forms, from other foods ingested by the child, requiring the addition of iron supplementation in infant formulas to minimize this difference.

Zinc also presents differentiated absorption, and its bioavailability in human milk is high, reaching 41% absorption against 28% in bovine milk, 31% in formulas and 14% in soy-based formulas, being necessary the addition during the manufacture of infant formulas (JOHNSON; EVANS, 1978). As well as multiple vitamins to meet the needs of newborns (ESCOBAR et al., 2002).

2.3 SURVEYED MICROBIOTA

2.3.1 Aerobic mesophilic micro-organisms

The group of total mesophilic aerobic microorganisms encompasses heterotrophic aerobic microorganisms whose optimum growth temperature range is 30 - 40°C (APHA, 2015).

The FAO states that the total mesophilic count should be applied to the finished product or any other point that provides information necessary for verification purposes. The safe production of these products depends on maintaining a high level of hygienic control, and the employment of additional microbiological criteria is a matter for the manufacturer as a means of ongoing assessment of their hygiene programmes, and not by the competent authority. The proposed criteria for aerobic mesophilic bacteria are reflective of Good Manufacturing Practices (GMP), providing useful indications of the hygienic status of processing steps (FAO, 2008; NATIONAL RESEARCH COUNCIL, 1985). With increased counts beyond recommended limits being indicative of bacterial accumulation in equipment such as evaporators or contamination due to leaks in plate heat exchangers (ibid)

For foods that undergo heat treatment, the analysis of this group has great relevance when no results are found for more specific analyses for pathogenic microorganisms, because even if no pathogenic microorganisms have been found in a sample, a high count of aerobic mesophilic microorganisms is indicative that the food may be unsuitable for consumption (APHA, 2015).

In a non-perishable food such as powdered infant formula, the high count of this group of microorganisms indicates the use of contaminated raw material or an inadequate processing from the hygienic-sanitary point of view. After re-suspension of infant formulas, these become perishable foods and this count indicates contamination during preparation or time conditions and inadequate storage temperature (BEUCHAT et al., 2013; FRANCO; LANDGRAF, 2003;).

2.3.2 Enterobacteriaceae

Enterobacteriaceae are facultative aerobic and anaerobic Gram negative bacilli that belong to the family *Enterobacteriaceae*. Although they have a ubiquitous distribution, most of them inhabit the intestines of humans and animals, either as members of the normal microbiota or as pathogens. The main genera in this group are *Escherichia, Shigella, Salmonella and Enterobacter* (FRANCO; LANDGRAF, 2003).

The presence of any member of the *Enterobacteriaceae* family is undesirable in pasteurized products. The method for total enterobacteriaceae count has greater sensitivity to detect post-processing contamination than the coliform count test, in addition to being faster and encompassing non-lactose fermenting pathogenic microorganisms (APHA, 2015).

2.3.3 Bacteria of the coliform group

The coliform group is composed of Gram negative, aerobic and facultative aerobic bacilli, non sporulated, belonging to the Enterobacteriaceae family and capable of fermenting lactose with acid and gas production. This group is formed by two groups, total coliforms and thermotolerant coliforms, being referred to by ANVISA as coliforms at 35°C and coliforms at 45°C, respectively (APHA, 2015; BRASIL, 2001).

The group of total coliforms are those capable of fermenting lactose when incubated at 35°C for 48 hours, being formed by more than 20 species including bacteria from the gastrointestinal tract of humans and warm-blooded animals (APHA, 2015; SILVA; JUNQUEIRA; SILVEIRA, 1997). The presence of total coliforms in a sample does not necessarily indicate the presence of pathogenic microorganisms. The group of thermotolerant coliforms are so named because they ferment lactose when incubated at a temperature range of
44,5 - 45.5°C for 24 hours. The main genera that compose the group are *Escherichia, Enterobacter and Klebsiella, Escherichia coli* being the main representative of the group and the only one which has as its natural habitat the intestine of humans and other warm-blooded animals, thus being directly related to contaminations of faecal origin (ibid).

The count of Enterobacteriaceae, coliforms and *E. colipermis allows us to* evaluate the overall quality of a food or the hygienic-sanitary conditions present during food processing. The presence of microorganisms of these groups in products submitted to heat treatment may indicate inefficiency in the pasteurization process or occurrence of post-processing contamination (FRANCO; LANDGRAF, 2003).

2.3.4 Coagulase positive Staphylococcus

Staphylococcus are Gram-positive, facultative anaerobic cocci, non-sporulated, immobile, capable of forming small rows or clumping together in grape cluster-like formations. They do not usually produce a capsule (SCHLEIFER; BELL, 2015).

The most studied species is *Staphylococcus aureus,* commonly found in humans and animals, colonizing the skin and nasal mucosa, but without causing damage to healthy carriers, responsible for most of the poisonings caused by ingestion of contaminated food. Other species of the genus *Staphylococcus* have been highlighted as potential opportunistic pathogens, especially in immunocompromised patients (GERMANO; GERMANO, 2011).

Staphylococcus have a very wide temperature range, ranging from 7-48°C, and are destroyed in products that are subjected to heat treatment. The presence of *Staphylococcus* in the final product occurs due to failures in technological processing or post-processing contamination (ICMSF, 1996; STEWART, 2003).

Bacterial multiplication leads to the risk of producing toxic compounds, all of which are heat-resistant and fast-acting in the gastrointestinal tract, compromising or not the overall appearance of the product (CDC, 2018).

The prevention of *Staphylococcus* growth in food is based on hygiene measures controls, including control of raw materials, proper handling, cleaning and disinfection of equipment. These practices are generally not sufficient to prevent or reduce its occurrence and proliferation in food products, requiring the combination with other treatments to prevent this proliferation (HENNEKINNE et al., 2012).

Due to the thermal processing employed, the presence of *Staphylococcus* in infant formulas occurs sporadically in infant formulas due to post-processing contaminations or during the handling of the product for consumption (BUCHANAN; ONI, 2012). Since these bacteria are colonizers of the skin, mouth and nose of handlers (TRABULSI; ALTERTHUM, 2008).

2.3.5 *Bacillus cereus*

The genus *Bacillus* is composed of Gram positive, aerobic or facultative aerobic rods. Some species have motility, toxin production and the ability to form spores. They occur singly, in pairs or in chains and are usually associated with soil, but can also be found in water and food. They cause foodborne diseases and opportunistic infections and produce spores resistant to heat, radiation and desiccation, compromising contaminated food (LOGAN; VOS, 2015). Among the species belonging to the genus, *Bacillus cereus* stands out, often associated with cereals and farinaceous, and producer of toxins capable of causing deterioration in food due to the production of enzymes (REIS, 2012). The microorganism can multiply in a pH range between 4.3-9.3. Most strains are mesophilic, with an optimum growth temperature between 25 and 37°C, but some strains have psychrotrophic characteristics (SCHOENI; WONG, 2005).

B. cereus is widely distributed in nature and is related to outbreaks of illness caused by different toxins: diarrhoeal syndrome and emetic syndrome. The emetic syndrome is characterised by signs and symptoms related to emesis and is caused by thermostable toxins in the food shortly after ingestion. However, the diarrheal form, whose main symptom is diarrhea, is associated with thermolabile toxins and takes a longer period to manifest itself (FORSYTHE, 2002; TRABULSI; ALTERTHUM, 2008).

The control of *B. cereus* contamination *in* food is very complicated, especially in the dairy industry. The main factors that hinder the elimination of *B. cereus* in the industry are the difficulty in obtaining raw milk free of *B. cereus,* due to the wide distribution in nature and the capacity of formation of spores, which are capable of resisting drastic thermal treatments and other stress conditions, besides strongly adhering to the surfaces of utensils and equipment (ANDERSSON et al., 1995). The presence of spores is of special importance in sterilized milk, acting as a deteriorant due to the capacity of producing enzymes that alter the sensory characteristics of the product (ORDÓNEZ, 2005; REIS, 2012).

The presence of *B. cereus* spores in the handling environment of a dairy is critical. Once the sample is contaminated with spores, the *B. cereus* can return to its vegetative form after reconstitution using heated water, and should be consumed as soon as possible to avoid increasing the microbial count. Due to the fragility of the age group to which this product will be offered, the whole process and its control should be performed according to good manufacturing practices and since the presence of *B. cereus*, even in small quantities, represents a risk of food toxinfection due to bacterial multiplication caused by inadequate storage (REZENDE-LAGO et al., 2007).

2.3.6 *Enterococcus* spp.

The genus *Enterococcus* is composed of Gram-positive, facultative aerobic cocci that are resistant to stress, do not produce spores and are generally catalase negative. Studies indicate the presence of hemolytic activity, but there is great variation among species (SVEC; DEVRIESE, 2015).

For many years, the genus has been employed in fermentative technologies in the food area, being used as probiotic. However, recently, the genus *Enterococcus has* stood out as a pathogen for humans, although the virulence factors are not fully elucidated. The species *E. faecalis,* considered the most pathogenic of the genus, and *E. faecium* are most commonly found in the human gastrointestinal tract, followed by the species *E. avium* and *E. hirae.* The increased pathogenicity of the genus is due to the development of antimicrobial resistance, the strains are resistant to several antimicrobials, including vancomycin (KAARME et al., 2015; NES; DIEP; IKE, 2014; SOARES-SANTOS; BARRETO; SEMEDO-LEMSADDEK, 2015).

2.3.7 Lactic acid bacteria

The lactic acid bacteria group is composed of Gram-positive bacteria, of varied morphology, mesophilic, generally immobile and non-spore forming, of different genera, facultative anaerobes or microaerophiles, whose main characteristic of this group is their ability to ferment glucose, a by-product of the breakdown of lactose, the main milk sugar, producing lactic acid. They are also capable of producing several antimicrobial factors, such as organic acids, hydrogen peroxide, nisins and bacteriocins (FORSYTHE, 2002; OLIVEIRA, 2009).

Lactic acid bacteria are widespread in nature, even in environments unfavourable to growth. They are used for fermented foods, meats, vegetables, beverages, fruits and as probiotics, and can also be found as constituents of the respiratory and gastrointestinal tracts, as well as in the cavities of humans and animals. Industrially, fermentation by lactic acid bacteria also helps in food preservation by producing antibacterial agents and acidifying the medium (OLIVEIRA, 2009).

However, the presence of lactic acid bacteria can also be harmful when it causes a reduction in the pH, resulting from the accumulation of lactic acid produced, leading to the precipitation of casein in raw milk (ORDÓNEZ, 2005).

This group includes the genera *Pediococcus, Streptococcus, Lactococcus, Leuconostoc, Lactobacillus* and *Bifidobacterium* (FORSYTHE, 2002; OLIVEIRA, 2009).

2.3.8 *Salmonella* spp.

Microorganisms of the genus *Salmonella* are Gram negative bacilli belonging to the family Enterobacteriaceae, facultative anaerobes and do not form spores. They are capable of producing hydrogen sulfide (H2S) and most have as their main reservoir the gastrointestinal tract of homeothermic animals, with some serovars being strictly species-specific (ICMSF, 1998; POPOFF; LE MINOR, 2015).

The concentration necessary to cause complications to humans depends on certain factors, such as the *Salmonella* serotype, the susceptibility of the individual and the type of food involved. Bacterial cells have the characteristic of being surrounded by globules of fat, which is a risk when thinking about foods with a high lipid content. This characteristic makes the bacteria resistant to stomach pH and the action of enzymes (ICMSF, 1998).

One of the most important vehicles of transmission of *Salmonella* spp. related to pathogenicity in humans is chicken meat. The symptoms of infection caused by *Salmonella* spp. involve gastrointestinal complications, such as diarrhea and colic, and fever, and may last for up to seven days, but do not require hospitalisation. However, individuals with low immunity may develop a more severe condition with the spread of the bacteria to other systems, possibly leading to death (CDC, 2015).

Contamination by *Salmonella* spp. can occur at any stage of food preparation. Failures in food storage, flaws in handling, increase in the trade of ready meals and increased consumption of raw food or subjected to inefficient heat treatment are factors identified as responsible for the increase in cases of salmonellosis (EVANGELISTA, 2009).

2.3.9 *Cronobacter sakazakii*

Cronobacter sakazakii, formerly *Enterobacter sakazakii,* is a Gram negative, facultative aerobic, opportunistic rod-shaped pathogen that is generally mobile and has a wide growth temperature and pH range. They are capable of biofilm formation and have resistance to heat, ultraviolet radiation, stomach acids, pasteurization due to the ability to produce a heteropolysaccharide capsule, and various antimicrobials. Outbreaks caused by the micro-organism are usually associated with dehydrated infant formula, but other foods have been linked to cases of the disease. Cases of infection have been reported in both children and the elderly, however, the mechanisms of pathogenicity and virulence have not yet been elucidated (FAKRUDDIN et al., 2013; IVERSEN et al., 2008; IVERSEN; FORSYTHE, 2003; KALYANTANDA, SHUMYAK and ARCHIBALD, 2015).

Several hospital infection outbreaks involving newborn babies have presented *C. sakazakii* as the etiologic agent and most have related infant formula powders and powdered milk as the sources of contamination (ACKER et al., 2001; CLARK et al., 1990; LEHNER and STEPHAN, 2004).

The Brazilian legislation does not contain maximum limits for the presence of this pathogen in this type of food (BRASIL, 2001). According to Franco (2012), this bacterium is considered an emerging agent and capable of major harm to consumer health. As for international standards, the FDA and the European Community establish that, in infant formulas, the required standard is the absence of *C. sakazakii* (EUROPEAN COMMUNITY, 2005; FDA, 2019).

2.3.10 **Mycobiota**

Fungi are capable of developing in various types of environment, and may be present in water, soil, debris and living beings such as humans and animals. Multiplication can occur both sexually and asexually, depending on the species, and dispersal occurs in nature by animals, water and especially wind, increasing their distribution. They are mostly saprophytes, consuming organic matter found in the soil, however, they can also be associated with canned food, in the form of spores, besides a whole range of utensils objects used for food handling (OLIVEIRA, 2014; TRABULSI; ALTERTHUM, 2008).

Most of the fungi considered pathogenic are related to the soil (TRABULSI; ALTERTHUM, 2008). Regarding resistance, both filamentous fungi and yeasts are able to develop in environments with lower water activity and lower pH levels (4.5 to 6.0 for yeasts and 3.5 to 4.0 for filamentous fungi) when compared to bacteria (FORSYTHE, 2002; GERMANO; GERMANO, 2011).

Fungal virulence factors are not very well elucidated, being usually attributed to genetic variety, ability to adhere to surfaces and the production of toxins and enzymes. There is also the capacity of synergistic relations with other microorganisms, which favours fungal development (TRABULSI; ALTERTHUM, 2008).

Fungal contamination is often found in foods with low water activity, such as powdered foods, especially foods rich in proteins and carbohydrates. Filamentous fungi have the potential to spread by conidia, which confer resistance to environmental adversities and extreme temperatures. Thus, products with disinfection potential, such as those employed in asepsis and disinfection of utensils used in handling, often have no effectiveness in controlling fungal conidia (MOURA et al., 2014; SANTOS et al., 2014).

The presence of fungi in hospital environments constitutes a serious risk to patients, since many are debilitated. The ventilation system of hospital units constitutes an excellent source of fungal contamination due to inefficient cleaning of the system as a whole and of the filters used in the air outlets. Air conditioning trays are pointed out as the main source of contamination in these environments presenting *Aspergillus* sp. and *Penicillium* sp. as the most frequent fungal contaminants (AFONSO et al., 2004; MARTINS-DINIZ et al. 2005; MOBIN; SALMITO, 2006; QUADROS et al., 2009).

The production of fungal toxins, mycotoxins, is observed in products of both plant and animal origin and can be detected at all levels of the food chain and are secondary metabolites produced mainly by the genera *Aspergillus, Fusarium* and *Penicillium* (FORSYTHE, 2002).

Xerophilic fungi are known to grow in environments with reduced water activity independent of other growth factors (PITT, 1998). The ease of fungi to develop in foods with low aqueous activity (Aa), the production of conidia and the ability of powdered supplements to reabsorb moisture from the environment are also factors of great importance, especially when considering the population group for whom the food supplements analysed are intended (FAO, 2006).

Among the xerophilic fungi, there is a group called moderate xerophilic, which is able to grow in a medium with low water activity and does not require specific medium for growth. In this group we can highlight species of the genera *Aspergillus* and *Penicillium* (SAMSON, 2002).

2.4 CHEMICAL CONTAMINANTS

2.4.1 **Mycotoxins**

The *Aspergillus* genus is worldwide associated with the production of toxins, especially in regions with warmer climates. Contamination generally occurs due to failures in the harvest and storage of products of vegetable origin, leading to the proliferation of the fungus and the production of the toxins, aflatoxin B1 and B2, the latter in lower concentration. When the products are used in the manufacture of animal feed, the aflatoxin B1 present is biotransformed in the ruminant liver and excreted in the milk as aflatoxin M1 (AFM1), capable of producing acute toxic and carcinogenic effects in several animal species. There is the possibility of AFM1 binding irreversibly to milk casein, resisting pasteurization and other processes for the production of dairy products, thus being transmitted to humans (GERMANO; GERMANO, 2011).

Ingestion of products contaminated with fungi and mycotoxins can lead to toxigenic disease. Acute cases are associated with kidney or liver damage, while prolonged exposure is associated with liver cancer. There is also the possibility of the occurrence of mutagenic alterations due to DNA damage and teratogenic, resulting in childhood cancer during the embryonic period (FORSYTHE, 2002; TRABULSI; ALTERTHUM, 2008).

The care with AFM1 should start from the initial quality of the sample since this toxin is thermo resistant, surviving at elevated temperatures as demonstrated by Iha et al. (2013) in which AFM1 concentrations were found in a range of 20 - 760ng/kg in 100% of the UHT and powdered milk samples evaluated.

The RDC n° 07 of 2011 (2011b) determines the maximum limit of aflatoxin M1 in fluid milk of 0.50pg/kg of the final product. This determination is being written along the lines of the values determined by the European community in which concentrations of 0.05pg/kg or L of AFM1 in infant formulas are provided, where there is knowledge of the dangers associated with the ingestion of mycotoxin (EUROPEAN COMMUNITY, 2006).

In light of the knowledge about these risks, several authors have been pointing out over the years the need for increased precaution and control of mycotoxins globally in order to minimize this intake (ALVITO et al., 2010; MEUCCI et al., 2009; TONON; SAVI; SCUSSEL, 2018).

2.4.2 Antimicrobial residues

Antimicrobials are compounds that reduce or inhibit microbial growth when used at optimal inhibitory concentrations. Antimicrobials can be divided into antibiotics and chemotherapeutics, antibiotics being substances naturally produced by fungi, yeasts or other microorganisms and chemotherapeutics being chemical substances produced by synthesis (Carneiro, 2011). Antimicrobials are important drugs used in human and veterinary medicine. In the field of veterinary medicine, antibiotics are used for therapeutic treatment of infections, prophylactic use for the prevention of diseases before or after exposure to it, and as feed additives to promote animal growth. They are widely used in all phases of production, or life cycle of animals, especially in infections of the mammary gland (mastitis) and in diseases of the respiratory tract (BUZALSKI; REYBROECK, 1997; SHAO et al., 2009).

Mitchell et al. (1998), stated that theoretically, all routes of antimicrobial administration lead to the appearance of residues in food of animal origin. Therefore, several of the residues present in the body of animals can be transferred to the population through milk and milk products. The concentrations found in the milk secretion may vary and can be attributed to several factors such as: the classes of antimicrobials, the type of formulation of the antimicrobial applied, the variations between species, the pH difference between blood plasma and milk, the amount of milk produced and the grace period (NASCIMENTO; MAESTRO; CAMPOS, 2001; SHAO et al., 2009). Being this presence frequently reported in the literature (BANDO et al., 2009; BERENDSEN et al., 2010; LOPEZ et al., 2008; RODRIGUES; DALL'AGNOLB;

BITTENCOURTA, 2012; TROMBETE; SANTOS; SOUZA, 2014).

According to Netto et al. (2005), in Brazil, the p-lactam class is the class of antimicrobials most used in the treatment of infections in dairy cows. The residues generated by the administration of these drugs may be dangerous to the health of consumers. They can cause allergic and toxic reactions, in the short term in some sensitive individuals, and in the long term, can result in chronic toxic effects or the development of antibiotic resistant bacteria in humans (BANDEIRA et al., 2014; GASTALHO; SILVA; RAMOS, 2014; GOMES; DEMOLY, 2005; RAISONPEYRON, 2001; SILVA; HOLLENBACH et al., 2010; SILVA; TEJADA; TIMM, 2014).

2.5 DETECTION OF CHEMICAL CONTAMINANTS

2.5.1 Screening methods

In order to perform screening analysis on the suspect samples, simple and easy to perform methodologies are used, such as Thin Layer Chromatography (TLC) and ELISA techniques (Enzyme Linked Immuno-Sorbent Assay) for the detection of mycotoxins. Although these techniques are very sensitive and can give a quantitative result for the detection of the analytes in question, they are commonly used as screening methodologies where the presence or absence of mycotoxins is evaluated qualitatively (WHO, 2001).

The CCD technique consists in placing on a chromatographic plate a spot of the sample to be evaluated and, in parallel, a spot of a standard analyte previously solubilized in solvent. After the procedure, the plate is eluted with another solvent mixture and, after drying, the plate is placed in an ultraviolet chamber in which it will be possible to evaluate the fluorescence of the runs and calculate the retention factor (RF) of the samples. The presence of a mycotoxin is confirmed if the sample has the same RF as the standard (SHUNDO; SABINO, 2006). The quantification of mycotoxins in the sample must be done by the recovery methodology described by SCOTT (1997).

Despite being a relatively easy technique to perform and routinely employed, the number of publications using CCD has decreased over time, as information on its use and data has not been published (SHUNDO; SABINO, 2006 apud TRUCKNESS, 2001) [1].

ELISA is a technique based on the principle of specific interaction between antibody and antigen. The technique consists of two steps, the first being the reaction between the antibody and the antigen and the second the revelation of the reaction by the enzymatic hydrolysis that occurs between the antigen-enzyme complex and the substrate (ZHENG; RICHARD; BINDER, 2006).

The World Health Organization indicates the ELISA as a screening test in food of animal and vegetable origin (WHO, 2001). The ELISA is a technique of low cost and easy execution, not requiring skilled labour. Its use in food quality control analyses contributes to the optimization of the aflatoxin detection process thanks to the sensitivity, specificity and speed of the method (WHO, 2001; ZHENG; RICHARD; BINDER, 2006).

ZHENG et al. (2006) also described that the ELISA is effective in the detection of concentrations above 2.5ppb. However, with the high incidence of false-positive results, low reproducibility, variation of results from 30 to 300% and the possibility of false-negative results described by AMARAL and JUNIOR (2006), it has been recommended the use of confirmatory techniques, such as chromatography to confirm the positive results of the ELISA test.

Regarding milk origin matrices, OLIVEIRA; GERMANO (1996) evaluated the efficiency of the ELISA technique in the quantification of aflatoxin M1 in powdered milk artificially contaminated after reconstitution and did not find significant variation between the added concentrations and the concentrations detected in the milk samples.

TRUCKSESS, M.W. *Rapid analysis (thin layer chromatographic and immunochemical methods) for mycotoxins in foods and feeds. In:* de Koe, W.J.; Samsom, R.A.; van Egmond, H.P.; Gilbert, J.; Sabino, M. (eds). Ponsen&Looyen, Wageningen, The Netherlands, 2001, p.29-40.

In another study, KIM et al. (2000), found no significant difference in the results obtained when analysing aflatoxin M1 levels in pasteurised milk, infant formula, milk powder and yoghurt, using ELISA and HPLC.

2.5.2 High performance liquid chromatography

The High Performance Liquid Chromatography (HPLC) is a separation technique that, due to the possibility of changes in the methodologies used, it is possible to make quantitative determinations with good sensitivity, besides the possibility of separating non-volatile and thermolabile species where gas chromatography cannot be used. As many compounds possess the mentioned characteristics, the field of application of HPLC is extremely vast.

HPLC is prominent in detections used by the pharmaceutical industry, environmental determinations and monitoring of certain contaminants, becoming, in the last 30 years, one of the most used analytical methods for qualitative and quantitative purposes (TONHI et al., 2001).

The purpose of chromatography is to separate individually the various constituents of a mixture of substances for identification, quantification or to obtain a pure substance. The separation occurs by passing the sample through a stationary phase by means of a solvent that will act as mobile phase. After the sample is injected into the equipment, the sample components are distributed between the two phases according to their polarities and move more slowly than the mobile phase due to the attraction force exerted by the stationary phase. In the balance of these attraction forces mediated by polarity, the speed with which each component moves through the system is determined, generating a specific retention time pattern for each substance, which can then be identified (DENOBILE; NASCIMENTO, 2004).

Despite all the qualities presented by the technique, the ability to identify substances is limited. Errors may occur during the qualitative stage of the technique due to the chemical and structural characteristics of the substances analysed. Although the retention time is characteristic of a compound, several other compounds of similar polarity may have the same retention time under the chromatographic conditions employed, even though they have different characteristics. This will cause a co-elution between these compounds, with only one peak being identified with greater intensity

(FELTRIN et al., 2006).

Due to the limitations of liquid chromatography, the use of complementary techniques for identification has become necessary. The use of the technique of Mass Spectrometry (MS) has been coupled to liquid chromatography to overcome this deficiency, being employed in routine studies for confirmation of target compounds than determining the identity of unknown compounds of interest (LANÇAS, 2009). In the LC/MS system, the sample separated by HPLC is injected into the mass spectrometer by techniques of Ionization at ambient pressure (IPA), which generate few ions to help in determining the chemical structure of the analytes investigated, the ions in turn pass through an analyzer and the apparatus emits peaks relative to the mass of the ions allowing more accurate identification (ibid).

2.6 FACTORS INFLUENCING MICROBIAL GROWTH

2.6.1 Contamination during technological processing

One of the forms of contamination of infant formulas is due to failures during their processing, which can be attributed both to failures during the selection of raw materials and during the cleaning of equipment. The selection of low quality raw materials is directly linked to the count of microorganisms in the final product thus changing the final quality of the product. This associated with processing failures result in non-compliant food for consumption (SANTOS et al., 2014).

As for the sanitization of the equipment, the RDC No. 275 of 2002 says that the processes of sanitization are comprised of two stages: cleaning and sanitization. Since this is a closed system equipment, this cleaning system encompasses cleaning steps using physical methods with rinses with heated water, alternating with cleaning steps using chemical products with acidic, basic and sanitizing compounds (BRASIL, 2002).

Usually, closed system industrial dryers have self-cleaning systems that use physical methods and, due to the size of the equipment, make it impossible to apply chemical products for cleaning, which favours the formation of biofilm by microorganisms, causing the recurrent contamination of bacteria, such as *Staphylococcus* spp. species (FRIEDRICZEWSK et al., 2018; KASNOWSKI et al., 2010; SALIMENA, 2014) and fungi (REGINATO et al., 2014).

2.6.2 **Post-processing contamination**

The contamination of infant formulas during handling can generate numerous damages to the consumer's health, especially in hospital environments. Ineffective protocols of hygiene and disinfection of utensils used, associated to human failures are related to the increase of microbial count after manipulation. The use of poorly cleaned utensils contributes to an increase in the count of mesophilic aerobic heterotrophic bacteria, which can increase the initial contamination by up to two logarithmic cycles (ALMEIDA, 1998; ROSSI et al., 2010; SANTOS; TONDO, 2000; SANTOS et al., 2004).

The training of handlers is also vital for maintaining microbiological control in infant formulas. Nienov et al. (2009) in a study assessing the microbiological quality in infant formulas, investigated different shifts during the lactation routine and found a percentage of > 50% contamination by mesophilic aerobic heterotrophic bacteria in the samples assessed, demonstrating the role of handlers as potential propagators of pathogenic microorganisms.

In research conducted in Canada, Leal (2010) observed that knowledge about safe food was higher among trained handlers, reinforcing the importance and the positive outcome of a food safety training for employees of a food production unit.

Fungi are known as environmental contaminants. Therefore, the place where these samples are handled are also critical points to be analyzed for fungal counts. Due to the easy dispersion of these microorganisms and inefficient cleaning protocols, fungi can be found in closed ventilation systems adhered to the filters used, being biological indicators with a maximum limit of 7.50×10^2 CFU/m^3 (BRASIL, 2003b).

Martins-Diniz et al. (2005) evaluated the presence of fungi in hospital environments and obtained mean values of 3.33×10^3 CFU/m^3 in intensive care units, values much higher than those recommended by the Brazilian legislation. Other studies also showed high values of fungal contamination in hospital environments, mainly pointing out the air conditioning system tray as the main source of microbial proliferation and the genera *Aspergillus* sp. and *Penicillium* sp. as the most frequent fungal contaminants (AFONSO et al., 2004; MOBIN; SALMITO, 2006; QUADROS et al., 2009).

2.6.3 **Thermal inactivation during handling**

Despite the thermal processing used, infant formulas are still subject to microbial contamination after their reconstitution due to external sources of contamination or sporulation of microorganisms resistant to technological processing. The possibility of microbial growth after rehydration, is a fact that should be considered in the consumption of infant formulas, especially when the product is not subjected to heating after preparation (BEUCHAT et al., 2013).

Therefore, the use of heated water during the re-suspension of infant formulas is important to reduce the microbial count. Kim and Park (2007) evaluated the presence and term resistance of *C. sakazakii* in infant formulas and found no significant reduction when heated water at 50°C was added. However, the increase in the temperature of the diluent was able to increase the level of inactivation. The use of water at 60°C was sufficient to cause a reduction of 1 - 2 log CFU/g, when the application of water at 70°C was evaluated, the reduction in the concentration of *C. sakazakiif was* of 4 - 6 log CFU/g.

Further studies again demonstrated this microbial reduction, where the addition of water at 60°C was able to reduce 2 - 5 log CFU/g, thus proving the effectiveness of resuspension with water heated to at least 60°C (CHEN et al., 2009; OSAILI et al., 2009).

Kennedy et al. (2005) observed an average decimal reduction value of 4.8 at 6,6 min at 60°C when heated in broth. In another study, conducted in India, still point out the presence of *Staphylococcus aureus* strains in foodborne outbreaks extremely heat resistant, with D values at 60°C > 15 min in broth (NEMA et al. 2007).

Montanari et al. (2015) in their studies still managed to isolate strains of several *Staphylococcus* species with the ability to survive at 80°C, until then not discovered and characterised.

Similarly to bacteria, the addition of hot water to the samples was sufficient to cause the inactivation or sporulation of fungi until the sample was again in favourable conditions for growth as evidenced by Marroni et al. (2009).

Doyle and Marth (1975) in their studies demonstrated that conidia of species of the genus *Aspergillus* are inactivated when submitted to a temperature range of 45 - 60°C. Other studies corroborate these data demonstrating the use of heating application at 60°C to inactivate fungi of the genus *Penicillium* (SHEARER et al., 2002; SALOMAO et al., 2009; GROOT et al., 2019).

3 **METHODOLOGY**

3.1 MATERIAL

The equipment, as well as most of the consumable material, necessary for the development of the research were available at the Laboratory of Microbiological Control of Products of Animal Origin of the Department of Food Technology of the Veterinary School of the Fluminense Federal University and at the State Center for Food Research and Quality (CEPQA) of the Agricultural Research Company of Rio de Janeiro (PESAGRO-RJ).

3.2 METHODOLOGY

3.2.1 **Obtaining the samples**

The samples of specific infant formulas for early childhood were provided by the milk bank of Hospital Universitário Antônio Pedro (HUAP) in the form of powdered supplement and its rehydrated form at two moments. A total of 36 samples were analysed, collected during 2019 with monthly intervals between them. Making a total of six lots, of two brands with market recognition, called sample X and sample Y, evaluated in three forms of presentation being them: formula in solid form, collected at the time of opening the primary packaging (T1); formula reconstituted in liquid form, at the time of sample reconstitution (T2) and formula reconstituted in liquid form, after 24 hours kept under refrigeration (T3). The samples were evaluated in duplicate samples.

The evaluated samples were collected aseptically using sterile tubes. The solid samples (T1) were collected in sterile centrifuge tubes open at the time of collection and the other samples (T2 and T3) in spouted bottles used by the lactatory to offer infant formulas, sterilized by autoclaving, as well as other utensils used in the handling and preparation of products. The samples were prepared following the HUAP operational handling protocols in order to correctly assess the quality of the products offered to patients. Sample T3 was kept under refrigeration in the

own dairy unit in order to evaluate the behaviour in the storage conditions of the unit.

As it is a powder product, it was not necessary to transport it under refrigeration, and the care was limited to avoiding mechanical damage and providing adequate storage as recommended by the manufacturers. The samples after resuspension were transported under refrigeration and immediately to the laboratory where the analyses were performed in order to maintain the characteristics of the samples. The T3 samples of each lot were transported under the same refrigeration conditions after the 24-hour period, and collected the day after the first collection.

Once obtained, the samples were transported to the Microbiological Control of Animal Products Laboratory of the Food Technology Department of the Veterinary School of the Fluminense Federal University, where the bacteriological analyses were performed. The fungus count and toxin extraction were performed in the State Center of Food Quality (CEPQA) in PESAGRO-RJ. The separation and identification of toxins and antibiotic residues were performed at the Laboratory of Mycology and Mycotoxins (LAMICO) at the Federal University of Minas Gerais.

3.2.2 Sample preparation

All samples were weighed on analytical scales in the safety zone provided by the Bunsen burner, obtaining samples of 25±0.2 grams in weight. To count total coliforms, *B. cereus,* coagulase positive *Staphylococcus, Enterococcus* and lactic acid bacteria, after weighing, the samples were diluted and homogenized, using 225mL of 0.1% peptone salt solution as diluent, thus obtaining the first dilution (10^{-1}). The same procedure was used to verify the presence of *Salmonella* spp. and *Cronobacter sakazakii,* but with 225mL and 450mL of 1% buffered peptone salt solution as diluent, respectively. All analyses were performed in analytical duplicate to minimize processing error.

3.2.3 Microbiological analyses

3.2.3.1 Bacteriological count and identification

For the bacteriological count and identification, the methodologies described in the "Compendium of Methods for the Microbiological Examination of foods" (APHA) were performed. The counts of total mesophiles (RYSER; SCHUMAN, 2015), *Bacillus cereus* (BENNET; TALLENT; HAIT, 2015), positive coagulase Staphylococcus

(BENNET; HAIT; TALLENT, 2015), *Salmonella* spp. (COX, et al, 2015), lactic acid bacteria (NJONGMETA et al., 2015) count of total coliforms, thermo tolerant and *Enterobacteriacaea* (KORNACKI; GURTLER; STAWICK, 2015). For the enumeration of the *Enterococcus* genus, the methodology according to MERCK (2002, modified by FRANCO, R.; MANTILLA, S., 2004) was performed and the research of *Cronobacter sakazakii;* by the modified ISO/TS 22964 method (ISO, 2006).

3.2.3.2 Enumeration and identification of fungi

For fungal count, serial decimal dilution was performed in plates (PITT; HOCKING, 1998). With inoculation of 0.1mL aliquots of each of the dilutions in two culture media: Dichloran Glycerol agar (DG18) for xerophilic fungi (PITT; HOCKING, 1998) and Dichloran Rose Bengal Chloramphenicol (DRBC) agar to estimate the total fungi (ABARCA et al., 1994). The plates were incubated at 25° C for seven days. All analyses were performed in analytical duplicate to minimize error in processing.

Extraction and analysis of residues and toxins

The samples were extracted using the modified QuEChERS based extraction method, following methodology described in the AOAC Official Methods of Analysis Manual (2007). All extractions were performed in duplicate to minimize analytical error. Sample screening was performed using commercial enzyme immunoassay kits for AFM1 (Aflatest®, *Vicam,* Watertown, MA, USA), following manufacturer's instructions. For quantification and analysis, evaluation was performed in a VICAM® Series-4EX fluorimeter (Watertown, MA, USA). AFM1 standards (5mg) were purchased from Sigma (St. Louis, MO, USA).

The stock solution (50pg/mL) and working solutions (2pg/mL) were prepared in methanol and their concentrations confirmed by UV light absorption using a Shimadzu UV-1201 spectrophotometer (Kyoto, Japan) (AOAC 2007), stored in amber flasks at -10°C for a period of three months. The limits of detection (LOD) and quantification (LOQ) were found by adding, decreasing, concentrations of the standard solution and submitted to extraction and quantification up to the lowest detectable concentration (LOD) and the lowest quantifiable concentration (LOQ), under suitable repeatability conditions (n = 5, RSD < 15%). The limits of detection and quantification found were

0.013pg/kg and 0.055pg/kg, respectively. .

3.2.6 Statistical analysis

The data analyses were performed by analysis of variance (ANOVA). Pearson's correlation and the T test were used to compare the data of enumeration of the different microorganisms in the different dairy supplements. As well as the Pearson test in the comparison of the data of contamination by mycotoxins, in the different formulations and comparisons between the times. The analyses were conducted using the PROC GLM computer program in SAS *(SAS Institute,* Cary, NC).

4 **RESULTS AND DISCUSSION**

4.1 RESULTS

After the evaluation of the 36 samples, lactic acid bacteria, *B. cereus, C. sakazakii,* coliforms, enterobacteriaceae, *Enterococcus* spp. and *Salmonella spp. were* not detected in any of the samples analysed. From the evaluations of the three evaluated times, of the different brands of infant formulas, the count values in CFU per gram of sample, are presented in the table below:

Table 1: Microbial count (CFU g^{-1}) for mesophilic aerobes (APC), coagulase positive *Staphylococcus*, filamentous fungi (DRBC) and xerophilic fungi (DG18) in infant formulae.

SamplesAPC	*Staphylococcus* coagulase positive	DRBCDG18
T1	5.0 x 102 ±1 .08 x 102 ± 1,25 x 102 a1 ,08 x 10^1 a	1.39 x 103 ±3 .38 x 103 ± 1,16 x 103 a 1,69 x 103 a
T2	4,46 x 102 ± < 1.0 x 10^1 b 4.38 x 102 b	5,17 x 102 ± 2,33 x 102 3.50 x 102 b ± 1.17 x 102 3,43 x 103
T3	9,93 x 103 ± 8.48 x 103 c < 1.0 x 10^1 c	5,33 x 102 ± ± 4.93 x 102 c 3,19 x 103

4.1.1 Counting of Mesophilic Microorganisms

From the total mesophil count (PCA), a maximum value of 1.84 x 10^4 CFU g^{-1} was obtained, and an average count value of 3.54 x 10^3 CFU g^{-1} . The minimum value coincides with the detection limit of the technique (1.0 x 10 CFU g$^{1-1}$).

The linear correlation test and Pearson's correlation was performed in order to evaluate the interrelation of the counts in the three evaluated times, for each sample. The test did not show significant correlation, for the index of 95% significance between the values in the proposed treatments (P=0.21). Complementarily, the degree of linear correlation between the points was evaluated and an r^2 = 0.35 was obtained, indicating no trend in the ratio of counts, indicative of distinct sources of contamination.

4.1.2 Coagulase positive *Staphylococcus*

The count of positive *Staphylococcus* coagulase had the maximum value of 2.17 x 102 CFU g^{-1} and an average value of 3.89 x 10 CFU g^{-1} . Since the limit established by Brazilian legislation is the total absence of microorganisms of this genus, some batches of samples are unsuitable for consumption.

By linear correlation between the points, an $r^2 = 0.30$ was obtained, suggesting no trend in the ratio of counts, and contamination by material handling. Pearson's correlation was not significant, for the index of 95% significance between the values of the proposed treatments (P=0.25).

4.1.3 Filamentous Fungi

From the filamentous fungi count (DRBC), we obtained a minimum value of 4.0 x 10 CFU g^{-1} , a maximum value of 2.55 x 10^3 CFU g^{-1} and a mean count value of 8.14 x 10^2 CFU g^{-1} , as shown in Table 1. From the identifications of genera and main species of filamentous fungi we have exposed in Table 2, the frequency distribution.

The linear correlation between the points showed an $r2 = 0.16$, with no tendency in the counts ratio, indicating diverse contamination sources among the counts. Pearson's correlation did not show significant correlation, for the index of 95% significance between the values in the proposed treatments (P=0,42).

4.1.4 Xerophilic Fungi

In the DG18 agar count, it was possible to observe a minimum value of 1.17 x 10^2 CFU g^{-1} , a maximum value of 6.61 x 10^3 CFU/g and an average value of 2.34 x 10^3 CFU g^{-1} .

In Pearson's correlation test, no significant correlation was observed among the analyzed plots (P=0.68), for the index of 95% significance. When evaluating the degree of linear correlation between the points had an $r2=0.67$ no trend was noted in the counts, suspecting various sources of contamination.

In the evaluation of frequency analysis, applied ANOVA, the T test was applied to compare the treatments and the difference between treatments was not significant for an index of 95% significance (P=0.23), being exposed in table 1.

Table 2: Absolute and percentage frequencies of fungal strains of the genera isolated in samples of newborn supplements.

Fungal genus	Absolute number in CFU	Frequency (%)
Total Fungal Load of Samples Evaluated		
Aspergillus sp.	21	26,58
Eurotium sp.	21	26,58
Penicillium sp.	19	24,05
Cladosporium sp.	6	7,59
Mucor sp.	6	7,60
Fusarium sp.	6	7,60
Total	79	100,0

Besides the counts, a great variety of fungi were also observed. The following genera were isolated: *Aspergillus, Cladosporum, Eurotium, Fusarium* and *Penicillium*. Among the *Aspergillus genus,* specimens of the species *A. flavus, A. fumigatus, A. ocracius, A. oryzae, A. parasiticus* and *A. niger were* found. Of the genus *Penicillium,* the species *P. citrinum, P. citronigrum, P. clavatus. From the genus Fusarium,* the species *P. verticillioides* and *P. solani* were isolated.

4.1.5 Developmental kinetic curve of micro-organisms

In figures 1 and 2 below, it was interpreted the counting curves in CFU g^{-1} , of the two analysed samples, in the three analyzed times: Initial (T1), after heat treatment (T2) and refrigerated after 24 hours of rehydration (T3).

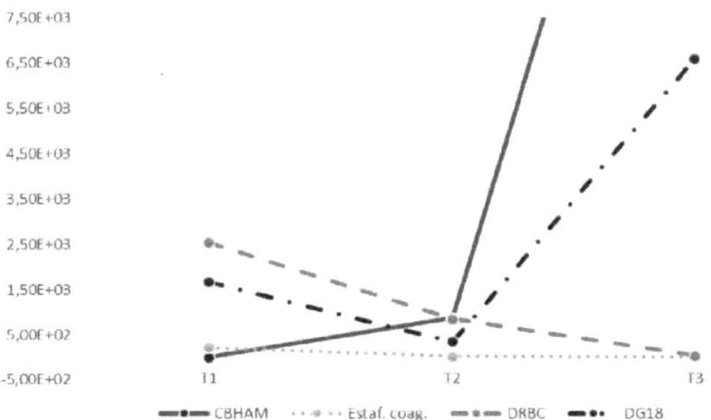

Figure 1: Counting curves of mesophilic bacteria (CBHAM), *Staphylococcus* (Staph. coag.), Filamentous Fungi (DRBC) and Xerophilic Fungi (DG18) at the times (T1, T2 and T3). - Sample X

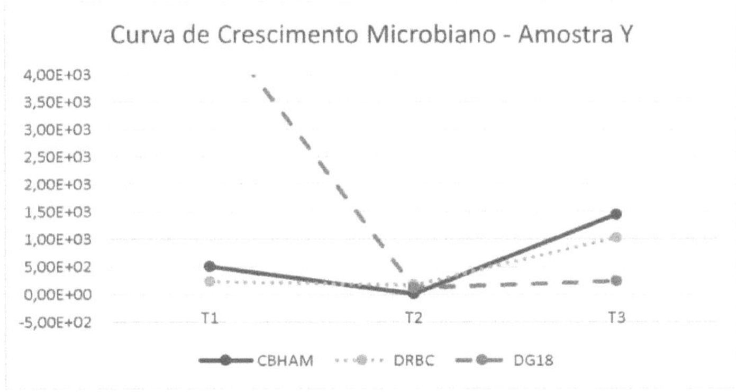

Figure 2: Counting curves of mesophilic bacteria (CBHAM), Filamentous Fungi (DRBC) and Xerophilic (DG18) at the times (T1, T2 and T3). - Sample Y

4.1.6 **Aflatoxin M1 analysis**

All the samples analysed remained below the detection limit of the technique as observed in Table 3:

Table 3: Mycotoxin concentrations (pg kg^{-1}) in infant formulae.

Samples	T1	T2	T3
X	<0,013	<0,013	<0,013
Y	<0,013	<0,013	<0,013

*LOD: <0.013 pg kg^{-1}

4.2 DISCUSSION

4.2.1 **Bacteriological Counting**

When analysing the two samples at the point of origin (T1), a significant difference was observed between the microbial count values. Sample X showed no count values for aerobic mesophiles while sample Y showed an initial count value of 5.0 x 10^2 CFU g .$^{-1}$

In Brazilian legislation there is no quality standard for mesophilic aerobic bacteria count in infant formulas. In comparison, the FDA has the "Compliance Program Guidance Manual" for the manufacture of infant formulas. In the manual, until 2018, the maximum limit for this type of microorganism in infant formulas was 10^4 CFU g^{-1} or mL^{-1}. Being used in the present study as a comparative factor for the evaluation of hygienic-sanitary quality, in which the formulas were handled (FAO, 2006).

Comparing the result of 5.0 x 10^2 CFU g^{-1} with the standard established by the FDA for CBHAM, it was observed that the count obtained was below that recommended in the manual. Despite the initial contamination, the sample is in conformity, being suitable for consumption.

Regarding the second point analyzed (T2), the two samples showed different behaviors when evaluating the growth curve of CBHAM. Because the reduction of the first point of curve T1, of sample Y, reached the detection limit count of the technique (< 1.0 x 10 CFU mL^{-1}). According to Kim and Park, 2007; Chen et al. , 2009; Osaili et al., 2009 this reduction is due to the addition of heated water for resuspension of infant formula causing damage to the cell structure and inactivation of viable cells. Beuchat et al., 2013 also pointed out the possibility of microbial growth after rehydration is a fact that should be considered in the consumption of food supplements, especially when the product is not heated after preparation.

According to the manufacturers' guidelines, water heated to at least 70°C must be used in the preparation of infant formulas, a temperature that is sufficient to cause microbial inactivation. This fact was corroborated by Kim and Park (2007) who evaluated the presence and thermo-resistance of *C. sakazakii* in infant formulas and found a reduction of 1 - 2 log CFU/g when using water at 60°C during resuspension and a reduction of 4 - 6 log CFU/g when using water at 70°C. Chen et al. (2009) and Osaili et al. (2009) in further studies found microbial reduction of 2 - 5 log CFU/g with the addition of water at 60°C thus proving the inhibitory effect observed in the present study.

When comparing the two brands studied, for brand X, figure 1, the inverse behaviour of sample Y was observed at the time evaluated (T2), with count values increasing, reaching higher values compared to T1 (8.83×10^2 CFU mL^{-1}), increasing exponentially until T3 (1.84×10^4 CFU mL^{-1}).

Buchanan; Oni 2012; and Reginato et al., 2014 stated that the increase in CBHAM count is indicative of unsatisfactory hygiene conditions in handling, with possible accumulation of bacteria in equipment used in the reconstitution of these formulas. Which leads to the assumption that the increase in the count of CBHAM of the analyzed samples occurs as described by the authors.

The contamination due to the handling of the samples is more evident in sample X observed in the parallel between the quality of the sample at T1 and the increase in the count at T2. However, when the samples were refrigerated for 24 hours after preparation, excessive growth of microorganisms was found in both samples (T3). Sample X had a count of 1.84×10^4 CFU mL^{-1} , figure 1, while sample Y remained below 1.50×10^3 CFU mL^{-1} , figure 2.

Despite the use of water at 70°C, the increased count of microorganisms can be attributed to the use of improperly cleaned utensils as observed by Almeida et al. (1998) who pointed the utensils used as one of the main causes of this contamination during the reconstitution of infant formulas in hospital settings, in which the count of CBHAM increased by up to two logarithmic cycles. Rossi et al. (2010), in subsequent studies, also evaluated the utensils used for the preparation of infant formulas and mean count values of 5.24 x 10^6 CFU g^{-1} were observed, evidencing the huge microbial load conveyed present in the utensils used in the preparation of these formulations reflected in the final count of 4.9 x 10^7 CFU g^{-1} or mL^{-1} of CBHAM in the infant formulas analyzed. Thus, corroborating the growth observed in the present work.

Another factor to be considered in this increase in the count of CBHAM is the handler with source of contamination, as evidenced by Santos et al. (2014) who evidenced count values above 5.8 x 10^7 CFU g^{-1} when analyzing the hands of handlers. Nienov et al. (2009) in a study evaluating the microbiological quality in infant formulas, investigated different shifts during the lactation routine and found a percentage of > 50% of contamination by mesophilic bacteria in the samples evaluated, proving the role of handlers can as potential propagators of pathogenic microorganisms.

Among the samples analyzed, it was observed in sample X the count for coagulase positive *Staphylococcus* (figure 1). At the first point analyzed (T1), a count of 2.17 x 10^2 CFU g^{-1} was observed, which decreased over time (T2 = 1.67 x 10 CFU mL^{-1}) until no detection at T3.

In the case of infant formulas of commercial recognition and established brand on the market, the count at the first point was found to be above the value permitted by Brazilian legislation, which recommends the total absence of this type of microorganism (BRASIL, 2001).

However, when comparing the analysis of total mesophiles and coagualase positive *Staphylococcus of* sample X, it can be said that the contamination occurred was due to handling failures as evidenced by Almeida et al. (1998) and Nienov et al. (2009). Buchanan and Oni (2012) pointed out that the mentioned microbiota occur only sporadically and at very low levels in infant formulas, as they are colonizers of the skin, mouth and nose of the manipulators. Santos et al. (2014) observed counts of up to 2.8 x 10^6 CFU g^{-1} when analysing the hands of the handlers. This corroborates the contamination observed in the present study.

When T2 was evaluated, it was again observed the reduction of microbial counts after the addition of water at 70°C for resuspension. This temperature is able to exponentially inhibit the growth of coagulase positive *Staphylococcus* as described by Kennedy et al (2005) in their study where a mean decimal reduction value of 4.8 to 6.6 min was observed at 60°C when heated in broth. The reduction value was pointed out by Nema et al. (2007) where extremely heat resistant strains of *Staphylococcus aureus* *were* found in foodborne outbreaks and D values at 60°C > 15 min were observed in broth.

4.2.2 **Fungal Count**

The growth of filamentous fungi (DRBC) presented the same pattern of behaviour in the two samples analysed as shown in figures 1 and 2.

The mycobiota, at the first analyzed points (T1) of each sample, showed high values for fungus count, 2.55 x 10^3 CFU g^{-1} for sample X (figure 1) and 2.33 x 10^2 CFU g^{-1} for sample Y (figure 2). Since the packages were opened at the time of collection, the initial contamination is may come from the raw material and handling during technological processing. Santos et al. (2014) attributed the contamination to both the inferior quality of the raw materials that make up the final product, as well as failures in the processing of the product.

The high counts as well as the variety of genera and fungal species found can be justified by the diversity of ingredients present in food supplements, each ingredient subject to contamination during its production, storage and transport.

Fungal contamination is often found in foods with low water activity, such as powdered foods, especially foods rich in proteins and carbohydrates (MOURA et al., 2014; SANTOS et al., 2014). Filamentous fungi have the potential to spread by conidia, which confer resistance such as: environmental adversities and extreme temperatures. Thus, products with disinfection potential, such as those employed in asepsis and disinfection of utensils used in handling, often have no effectiveness in controlling fungal conidia.

Fungi are known as environmental contaminants. Therefore, the place where samples are handled are also critical points to be analyzed for fungal counts. Due to the easy dispersion of these microorganisms and inefficient cleaning protocols, fungi can be found in closed ventilation systems adhered to the filters used, being biological indicators with a maximum limit of 7.50 x 10^2 CFU m^{-3} (BRASIL, 2003b).

Martins-Diniz et al. (2005) evaluated the presence of fungi in hospital environments and obtained mean values of 3.33 x 10^3 CFU m^{-3} in intensive care units, values much higher than those recommended by the Brazilian legislation. In other studies high values of fungal contamination were observed in hospital environments, considering mainly the air conditioning system tray as the main source of microbial proliferation and the genera *Aspergillus* spp. and *Penicillium* spp. as the most frequent fungal contaminants (AFONSO et al., 2004; MOBIN; SALMITO, 2006; QUADROS et al., 2009).

When analysed at the second time point (T2), a significant drop in the count was observed after adding hot water for resuspension of the samples, reaching values of 8.67×10^2 CFU mL^{-1} for sample X and 1.67×102 CFU mL^{-1} for sample Y, as shown in figures 1 and 2.

Similarly to bacteria, the addition of hot water to the samples was sufficient to cause the inactivation or the sporulation of fungi until the sample was again in favourable conditions for growth as evidenced by Marroni et al (2009). Doyle and Marth (1975) in their studies demonstrated that conidia of species of the genus *Aspergillus* are inactivated when submitted to a temperature range of 45° - 60°C. Solomon et al. (2009); Shearer et al. (2002); Groot et al. (2019) corroborated the results observed previously regarding the use of the application of heating at 60°C to inactivate fungi of the genus *Penicillium.*

When the third point was evaluated, the growth curve for filamentous fungi differed between the two samples. In sample X (Figure 1), the decline in the microbial concentration of filamentous fungi continues to be observed, caused by the inability to retake the filamentous form due to the addition of water and thus reducing the number of viable cells, reaching values close to zero. Based on the behavioral pattern of the growth curve, it can be stated that the contamination of sample X is mostly from failures during the manufacture of the product, a fact evidenced by inactivation.

While in sample Y (figure 2), there was an increase in relation to the previous count, obtaining a count of 1.03×10^3 CFU mL^{-1} . The contaminants in sample Y had a higher germination capacity than the other sample analysed, a fact that can be attributed to environmental contamination during handling, which introduced viable cells that were not so affected by the addition of heated water. These cells, despite having been inactivated at T2, did not suffer such severe cellular damage that allowed growth during the 24-hour storage period.

As for the analysis of xerophilic fungi (DG18), both samples were found high values in T1 (figures 1 and 2). In sample X a value of 1.68×10^3 CFU g^{-1} was observed while sample Y had higher count (5.07×103 CFU g^{-1}).

Xerophilic fungi are known to grow in environments with reduced water activity independent of other growth factors (PITT, 1998). It was considered that the initial mycobiota isolated comes from the sample itself. Thus, the quality of the raw materials used in their formulation should be controlled in order to avoid this contaminant load.

The way infant formulas are stored influences the fungal growth, as evidenced in the difference of count between the two distinct brands. The ease of fungi to develop in foods with low water activity (Aa), the production of conidia and the ability of powdered supplements to reabsorb moisture from the environment are also factors of great importance, especially when considering the population group for whom the food supplements analysed are intended (FAO, 2006).

The behaviour of the growth curve of the xerophilic fungi was the same as that of the filamentous fungi in T2, there being a decrease of one logarithmic cycle in the cell concentration of both samples due to the resuspension of the sample using water heated to 70°C, being similar to the data cited in the literature (DOYLE; MARTH, 1975; GROOT et al., 2019; SALOMAO et al., 2009; SHEARER et al., 2002).

As for the third time period analysed, the growth curves showed different behaviours among the brands in relation to the growth curve of filamentous fungi.

In sample X (figure 1) it can be observed that the growth of xerophilic fungi was quite high, with counts above 10^3 CFU mL^{-1} , while low counts of filamentous fungi were observed in the order of 10 CFU mL^{-1}

Although the sample contained high microbial load from manufacturing (T1), the exponential increase in growth is closely related to environmental contamination during the handling stage, given the drastic cell inactivation observed in T2.

Unlike sample X, in sample Y insignificant growth of xerophilic fungi was found at T3 (1.17 x10^2 CFU mL^{-1} at T2 and 2.38 x 102 CFU mL^{-1}). From the constancy in the cell count of sample Y throughout the last points analyzed, it can be stated that during the handling and storage of the resuspended sample, there was no environmental contamination as in the previous sample. The small growth at T3 was due to cells present at T1 whose functions were re-established after application of the heat treatment at T2.

Among the xerophilic fungi, there is a group called moderate xerophilic, which is able to grow in a medium with low water activity and does not require specific medium for growth. This group includes species of the genera *Aspergillus* and *Penicillium*

(SAMSON, 2002). The primary identification of the colonies found revealed members of the genera *Aspergillus* and *Penicillium,* thus confirming contamination due to ineffective control of sanitization of the air conditioning system, as described by other studies (AFONSO et al., 2004; MOBIN; SALMITO, 2006; QUADROS et al., 2009).

4.2.3 **Mycotoxin evaluation**

After performing the fluorimetric analyses, no AFM1 concentrations were found in the samples analysed at any of the three points analysed in the study, being below the detection limit as shown in Table 3.

In the Brazilian legislation, the maximum limit of AFM1 is 0.50pg kg^{-1} of the final product, and 100% of the samples analyzed were within the limits recommended by the legislation. Regarding international standards, the European Community (2006) mentions the concentration of 0.05pg kg^{-1} or L^{-1} of AFM1 in infant formulas.

The absence of mycotoxins in the samples evaluated in the present work are suggestive of the gradual increase in mycotoxin precaution and control globally as described by Alvito et al. (2010), Meucii et al. (2009) and Tonon, Savi and Scussel (2018).

Caution with AFM1 should start from the initial quality of the sample since the toxin is thermo resistant, surviving at elevated temperatures as demonstrated by Iha et al. (2013) in which AFM1 concentrations were found in a range of 20 - 760 ng kg^{-1} in 100% of the UHT and powdered milk samples evaluated.

5 CONCLUSION

The products analysed were in compliance with Brazilian legislation and with international standards in force. They are considered safe for consumption, but the need for immediate consumption after resuspension is reinforced in order to avoid undesirable microbial development.

Although the analyzed products were in conformity, the contaminations pointed out in this study indicate the need for greater efforts regarding the control of the manufacturing process of the products, whether they are the quality of the raw material used or the cleaning processes of the equipment used by the industry. Besides, the need for periodic training of professionals in the lactation units that will handle these products and the review of protocols for cleaning the utensils used.

6 BIBLIOGRAPHIC REFERENCES

ABARCA, M.L.; BRAGULAT, MR.; CASTELLA, G.; CABANES, P.J. Ochratoxin A production by strains of *Aspergillus niger var. niger*. *Applied and Environmental Microbiology*. v.60, p 2650-2652, 1994.

ACKER, J. V.; SMET, P.; MUYLDERMANS, G.; BOLGATEF, A.; LAUWERS, S. Outbreak of Necrotizing Enterocolitis Associated with *Enterobacter sakazakii* in Powdered Milk Formula. *Journal of Clinical Microbiology*, v. 39, n. 1, p. 293-297. 2001.

AFONSO, M. S. M.; TIPPLE, A. P. V.; SOUZA, A. C. S.; PRADO, M. A.; ANDERS, P. S. A qualidade do ar em ambientes hospitalares climatizados e sua Influência na ocorrência de infecções. *Revista Eletrónica de Enfermagem*, v. 6, n. 2, p. 181-188, 2004.

ALIJALOUD, S. O.; IBRAHIM, S. A.; FRASER, A. M.; SONG, T.; SHAHBAZI, A. Microbiological quality and safety of dietary supplements sold in Saudi Arabia. *Food Science and Nutrition*. v. 25. p. 593-596. 2013.

ALMEIDA, J.A.G.de; GOMES, R. Amamentação: um híbrido natureza-cultura. *Revista latino-americana de enfermagem*, v. 6, n. 3, p. 71-76. 1998.

ALMEIDA, R.C.C.; MATOS, C.O.; ALMEIDA, P.P. Implementation of a HACCP system for on-site hospital preparation of infant formula. Food Control. v.10, p.181-197, 1999.

ALVITO, P. C.; SIZOO, E. A.; ALMEIDA, C. M. M.; van EGMOND, H. P. Occurrence of Aflatoxins and Ochratoxin A in Baby Foods in Portugal. *Food Analitycal Methods*, v. 3, p. 22-30. 2010.

AMARAL, K. A. S. do; JUNIOR, M. M. Métodos analíticos para a determinação de aflatoxinas em milho e seus derivados: A review. *Revista Analytica*, Maringá, n. 24, p. 60-62, 2006.

ANDERSSON, A.; RÔNNER, U.; GRANUM, P.E. What problems does the food industry have with the spore-forming pathogens *Bacillus cereus* and *Clostridium perfringens*? *International Journal of Food Microbiology*. v.28, p. 145-155, 1995

AOAC. Association of Official Analytical Chemists. *Official Methods of Analysis* 19 ed. Gaithersburgh, Maryland: Association of Official Analytical Chemists International 2007.

APHA. AMERICAN PUBLIC HEALTH ASSOCIATION. *Compendium of Methods for the Microbiological Examination of foods*. 3 ed. Washington. 2015, 1219p.

AYTENFSU, S.; MAMO, G.; KEBEDEL, B. Review on Chemical Residues in Milk and Their Public Health Concern in Ethiopia. *Journal of Nutrition & Food Sciences*, v. 6, n 4. 2016.

BANDEIRA, M. G. L.; SANTOS, A. S.; ABRANTES, M. R.; REBOUÇAS, G. G.; SILVA, M . E. T.; PAIVA, W. S.; MAIA, M. O.; LIMA, L. S. C.; SILVA, J. B. A.; DAMACENO, M.

N . Sensitivity profile of Staphylococcus spp. isolated from food to antibiotics of pharmaceutical use. In: *Proceedings of the XII Latin American Congress on Food Microbiology and Hygiene.* Blucher Food Science Proceedings, v. 1, n. 1, p. 23-24, São Paulo, 2014.

BANDO, E.; OLIVEIRA, R. C.; FERREIRA, G. M.; MACHINSKI, M. Occurrence of antimicrobial residues in pasteurized milk commercialized in the state of Parana, Brazil. *Journal of Food Protection,* v. 72, p. 911-914, 2009.

BENNET, R. W.; HAIT, J. M.; TALLENT, S. M. *Staphylococcus aureus* and *Staphylococcal* enterotoxins in *Compendium of Methods for the Microbiological Examination of Foods,* 5 ed.

BENNET, R. W.; TALLENT, S. M.; HAIT, J.M. *Bacillus cereus* and *Bacillus cereus* toxins in *Compendium of Methods for the Microbiological Examination of Foods,* 5 ed.

BERENDSEN, B.; STOLKER, L.; DE JONG, J.; NIELEN, M.; TSERENDORJ, E.; SODNOMDARJAA, R.; CANNAVAN, A.; ELLIOTT, C. Evidence of natural occurrence of the banned antibiotic chloramphenicol in herbs and grass. *Analytical and Bioanalytical Chemistry,* v. 397, n. 5, p. 1955-1963, 2010.

BEUCHAT, L. R.; KOMITOPOULOU, E.; BECKERS, H.; BETTS, R. P.; BOURDICHON, P.; FANNING, S.; JOOSTEN, H. M.; KUILE, B. H. T. Low-Water Activity Foods: Increased Concern as Vehicles of Foodborne Pathogens. *Journal of Food Protection,* v. 76, n. 1, p. 150-172. 2013.

BRASIL. Ministry of Health. National Health Surveillance Agency (ANVISA). Resolution of the collegiate directory - RDC n° 12, of 2 January 2001. Aprova o regulamento técnico sobre padrões microbiológicos para alimentos, em anexo. *Diário Oficial [da] União,* Brasília, DF, n. 7, p. 45, 10 jan. 2001. Section 1.

BRASIL. Ministry of Health. National Health Surveillance Agency (ANVISA). Resolução da diretoria collegiada - RDC n° 275, de 21 de outubro de 2002. Aprovar o Regulamento Técnico de Procedimentos Operacionais Padronizados aplicados aos Estabelecimentos Produtores/Industrializadores de Alimentos e a Lista de Verificação das Boas Práticas de Fabricação em Estabelecimentos Produtores/Industrializadores de Alimentos. *Diário Oficial [da] União,* Brasília, DF, n. 206, p. 126, 23 oct. 2002. Section 1.

BRASIL. Ministry of Health. National Health Surveillance Agency (ANVISA). Resolution-RE no 9, 16 January 2003. Determines the publication of technical guidance prepared by a technical advisory group, on reference standards for indoor air quality in artificially conditioned environments of public and collective use. *Diário Oficial [da] União,* Brasília, DF, n. 114, p. 35, 20 jan. 2003, b. Section 1.

BRAZIL. Ministry of Agriculture and Supply. Normative Ruling No. 42, of 20 December 1999. Altera o Plano Nacional do Controle de Resíduos em Produtos de Origem Animal - PNCR e os Programas de Controle de Resíduos em Carne - PCRC, Mel - PCRM, Leite - PCRL e Pescado - PCRP. *Diário Oficial [da] União,* Brasília, DF, n. 181, p. 253, 22 Dec. 1999. Section 1.

BRASIL. Ministry of Health. National Health Surveillance Agency (ANVISA). Resolution of the collegiate board - RDC No. 253, of 16 September 2003. Cria o Programa de Análise de Resíduos de Medicamentos Veterinários em Alimentos de Origem Animal - PAMVet. *Diário Oficial [da] União,* Brasília, DF, n. 181, p. 90, 18 sep. 2003, a. Section 1.

BRASIL. Ministry of Health. National Health Surveillance Agency (ANVISA). Resolution of the collegiate directorate - RDC No. 44, September 19, 2011. Regulamento técnico para fórmulas infantis de seguimento para lactentes e crianças de primeira infância. *Diário Oficial [da] União,* Brasília, DF, n. 182, p. 92, 21 Sep. 2011, a. Section 1.

BRASIL. Ministry of health. Agência Nacional de Vigilância Sanitária. Resolução da diretoria collegiada- RDC n° 7, de 18 de fevereiro de 2011. Dispõe sobre limites máximos tolerados (LMT) para micotoxinas em alimentos. *Diário Oficial [da] União,* Brasília, DF, n. 7, p. 72, 22 fev. 2011b. Section 1.

BRASIL. Ministry of Health. National Agency of Sanitary Surveillance. Resolution of the collegiate directorate- RDC No. 243, of July 26, 2018. Dispõe sobre os requisitos sanitários dos suplementos alimentares. *Diário Oficial [da] União,* Brasília, DF, n. 144, p. 100, 27 jul. 2018. Section 1.

BRASIL. Ministry of Health. Anvisa. Agência Nacional De Vigilância Sanitária (ANVISA). *Program of Analysis of Residues of Veterinary Drugs in Food (PAMvet).* Report 2006-2007, 2009.

BRODY - Human Pharmacology. 4. ed. Rio de Janeiro: Elsevier, 2006.724p. Centers for Disease Control and Prevention. *E. coli homepage.* Revised Dec. 2014. Available at: < http://www.cdc.gov/ecoli/general/index.html>. Accessed 06 Apr. 2019.

BUCHANAN, R. L.; ONI, R. Use of Microbiological Indicators for Assessing Hygiene Controls for the Manufacture of Powdered Infant Formula. Journal of Food Protection, V. 75, N. 5, P. 989-997. 2012.

BUZALSKI, T. H.; REYBROECK, W. Antimicrobials. In: *International Dairy Federaltion standard (IDF/FIL).* Monograph on residues and contaminants in milk and milk products. Brussels: IDF, 1997. Special Issue, p. 26-34

CALIL V. M. L. T.; FALCÃO, M.C. Composição do leite humano: o alimento ideal. *Revista de Medicina,* v. 82, p. 1-10. 2003.

CARNEIRO, M.; FERRAZ, T.; BUENO, M.; KOCH, B. E.; FORESTI, C.; LENA, V. P.; MACHADO, J. A.; RAUBER, J. M.; KRUMMENAAUER, E. C.; LAZAROTO, D. M. The use of antimicrobials in a teaching hospital: a brief evaluation. *Revista da Associação Médica Brasileira,* v. 57, n. 4, p. 421-424. 2011.

CDC. Centers for Disease Control and Prevention. *Salmonella homepage.* Revised Apr. 2019. Available from:< http://www.cdc.gov/salmonella/index.html>. Accessed 26 Apr. 2015.

CDC. Centers for Disease Control and Prevention. Staphylococcal Food Poisoning In: *Food Safety Homepage.* Revised Aug. 2018. Available from:<

http://www.cdc.gov/foodsafety/diseases/staphylococcal.html >. Accessed 26 Apr 2019.

EC. EUROPEAN COMMUNITY. Regulation N° 2073/2005 of 15 November 2005 on microbiological criteria for foodstuffs. *Official Journal of the European Union,* 22 December 2005.

CHEN, P. C.; ZAHOOR, T.; OH, S. W.; KANG, D. H. Effect of heat treatment on *Cronobacter* spp. in reconstituted, dried infant formula: preparation guidelines for manufacturers. *Letters in Applied Microbiology,* v. 49, p. 730-737. 2009.

CLARK, N.C.; HILL, B.C.; O'HARA, C.M.; STEINGRIMSSON, O.; COOKSEY, R.C. Epidemiologic typing of *Enterobater sakazakii* in two neonatal nosocomial outbreaks. *Diagnostic Microbiology and Infectious Disease.* v.13, p.467-472. 1990.

CORTEZ, N. M. S.; CALIXTO, P. A. A.; CAMPOS, O. P. de; ZOCCAL, R.; FRANCO, R. M.; CORTEZ, M. A. S. Evaluation of production and bacteriological quality and detection of bacteriophages and antimicrobial agents in cheese whey produced in Rio de Janeiro state. *Revista Brasileira Ciência Veterinária.* v. 20. n. 3. jul./set. p. 166-171. 2013.

COX, N. A.; FRYE, J. G.; McMAHON, W.; JACKSON, C. R.; RICHARDSON, J.; COSBY, D. E.; MEAD, G.; DOYLE, M. P. *Salmonella* in *Compendium of Methods for the Microbiological Examination of Foods,* 5 ed., Washington: American Public Health Association, 2015, 985p.

COSTA, R. B. L; MONTEIRO, C. A. Consumo de leite de vaca e anemia na infância no Município de São Paulo. *Revista Saúde Pública,* v. 38, n. 6, p. 797-803. 2004.

CRUZ, D. C. S.; SUMAM, N. S.; SPÍNDOLA, T. Os cuidados imediatos prestados ao recém-nascido e a promoção do vínculo mãe-bebê. *Revista da Escola de Enfermagem USP,* v. 41, n. 4, p. 690-697. 2007.

DENOBILE, M.; NASCIMENTO, E. S. Validation of a method for determination of oxytetracycline, tetracycline, chlortetracycline and doxycycline antibiotic residues in milk by high performance liquid chromatography. *Revista Brasileira de Ciências Farmacêuticas,* v. 40, n. 2, p. 209-2018. 2004.

DILKIN, P. *Swine Mycotoxicosis:* Preventive, Clinical and Pathological Aspects. *Biológico,* 2002, 191p.

DOYLE, M. P.; MARTH, E. H. Thermal inactivation of conidia from *Aspergillus flavus* and *Aspergillus parasiticus. Journal of milk food technology,* v. 38, n. 11, p. 678-682. 1975.

EVANGELISTA, J. *Alimentos:* Um Estudo Abrangente. Rio de Janeiro: Atheneu. 2009.

ESCOBAR, A. M. U; OGAWA, A. R.; HIRATSUKA, M.; KAWASHITA, M. Y.; TERUYA, P. Y.; GRISI, S. Breastfeeding and socioeconomic cultural status: factors that lead to early weaning. *Revista Brasileira Saúde Materno Infantil,* v. 2, n. 3, p. 253-261.2002.

FAKRUDDIN, Md.; RAHAMAN, Md. M.; AHMED, M.M.; HOQUE, Md. M. *Cronobacter sakazakii (Enterobacter sakazakii):* An Emerging Foodborne Pathogen. *International*

Journal of Biomedical And Advance Research. v.4, n.6, 2013.

FAO. FOOD AND AGRICULTURE ORGANIZATION OF UNITED NATIONS. CAC/GL 55, *Guidelines for vitamin and mineral food supplements*. Rome. 2005.

FAO. FOOD AND AGRICULTURE ORGANIZATION OF UNITED NATIONS. CAC/RCP 66, *Code of hygienic practice for powdered formulae for infants and young children*. Rome, 2008.

FAO/WHO Food and Agriculture Organization of the United Nations/World Health Organization. General Standard for contaminants and toxins in food and feed CXS 1931995. 2014. 65p.

FDA. TITLE 21 - FOOD AND DRUGS, CHAPTER I - FOOD AND DRUGS ADMINISTRATION, DEPARTMENT OF HEALTH AND HUMAN SERVICES, SUBCHAPTER B - FOOD FOR HUMAN CONSUMPTION. PART 106 INFANT FORMULA REQUIREMENTS PERTAINING TO CURRENT GOOD MANUFACTURING PRACTICE, QUALITY CONTROL PROCEDURES, QUALITY FACTORS, RECORDS AND REPORTS AND NOTIFICATIONS. Code of Federal Regulations. Title 21, volume 2, 21CFR106. Revised as of April 1,2018.

FDA. U.S. Department of Health and Human Service Food and Drug Administration. *Compliance Program Guidance Manual*. USA. 2006, 31. Food Composition, Standards, Labeling and Economics.31 July 2006.

FELTRIN, C. W.; MELLO, A. M. S.; SANTOS, J. G. R.; MARQUES, M. V.; SEIBEL, N. M.; FONTOURA, L. A. M. Quantification of sulfadimethoxin in milk by high performance liquid chromatography. *Química Nova,* v. 30, n. 1, p. 80-82. 2007.

FOMON S. J. Bioavailability of supplemental iron in commercially prepared dry infant cereals. *Journal of Pediatrics,* v. 110, n. 4, p. 660-661. 1987.

FORSYTHE, S. J. *Microbiologia da Segurança Alimentar.* Porto Alegre: Artmed, 2002. 422p.

FRANCO, B.D.G.M.; LANDGRAF, M. *Microbiologia de Alimentos.* São Paulo. Editora Atheneu, 2003, 182 p.

FRANCO, R. M. *Etiológicos Agentes de Doenças Alimentares.* Niterói: Editora UFF, 2012. 119p.

FRIEDRICZEWSKI, A. B., GANDRA, E. A.; CONCEIÇÃO, R. C. S.; CERESER, N. D.; MOREIRA, L. M.; TIMM, C. D. Formation of biofilm by *Staphylococcus aureus* isolated from mozzarella cheese made with buffalo milk and its effect on sanitizer sensitivity. *Acta Scientiae Veterinariae,* n. 46, v.1528, p. 1-6. 2018.

GASTALHO, S.; SILVA, G. J.; RAMOS, P. Antibiotic use in aquaculture and bacterial resistance: Impact on public health. *Acta Farmacêutica Portuguesa,* v. 3, n. 1, p. 29-45, 2014.

GERMANO, P. M. L.; GERMANO, M. I. S. *Higiene e Vigilância Sanitária de Alimentos.* 4. ed. São Paulo: Manole, 2011. 1034 p.

GOMES, E. R.; DEMOLY, P. Epidemiology of hypersensitivity drug reactions. *Current Opinion in Allergy and Clinical Immunology,* v. 5, p. 309-316, 2005.

GROOT, M. N.; ABEE, T.; VEEN, H. B. Inactivation of conidia from three *Penicillium* spp. isolated from fruit juices by conventional and alternative mild preservation technologies and disinfection treatments. *Food Microbiology,* v. 81, p. 108-114. 2019.

GUERRA, A.; RÊGO, C.; SILVA, D.; FERREIRA G. C.; MANSILHA, H.; ANTUNES, H.; FERREIRA, R. Alimentação e nutrição do lactente. *Acta Pediátrica Portuguesa,* v. 43, n. 5, p.1-32. 2012.

HENNEKINNE, J. A.; DE BUYSER, M. L.; DRAGACCI, SYLVIANE. *Staphylococcus aureus* and its food poisoning toxins: characterization and outbreak investigation. *FEMS Microbiology reviews,* p. 1 -22. 2011.

ICMSF INTERNATIONAL COMMISSION ON MICROBIOLOGICAL SPECIFICATIONS FOR FOODS *Staphylococcus aureus.* Ch 17 In: *Microorganisms in food: Microbiological specifications of food pathogens.* Blackie Academic and Professional, 5 ed, London. 1996. p. 299-333.

ICMSF. INTERNATIONAL COMMISSION ON MICROBIOLOGICAL SPECIFICATIONS FOR FOODS. *Microorganisms in food:* Characteristics of microbial pathogens. London: Blackie Academic & Professional, v.5. 1998. 513p.

IHA, M. H.; BARBOSA, C. B.; OKADA, I. A.; TRUCKSESS, M. W. Aflatoxin M1 in milk and distribution and stability of aflatoxin M1 during production and storage of yoghurt and cheese. *Food Control,* v. 29, p. 1-6. 2013.

INNIS, S. M.; DYER, R.; NELSON, C. M. Evidence That Palmitic Acid Is Absorbed as sn-2 Monoacylglycerol from Human Milk by Breast-Fed Infants. *Lipids,* v. 29, n. 8, p. 541-545. 1994.

ISO. INTERNATIONAL ORGANIZATION FOR STANDARDIZATION.ISO/TS 22964:2006(E). *Milk and Milk products* - Detection of *Enterobacter sakazakii.* 2006.

IVERSEN, C.; FORSYTHE, S. J. Comparison of Media for the Isolation of *Enterobacter sakazakii. Applied and Environmental Microbiology.* v. 73. n. 1, p. 48-52. 2006.

IVERSEN, C.; MULLANE, N.; MCCARDELL, B.; TALL, B. D.; LEHNER, A.; FANNING, S .; STEPHAN, R.; JOOSTEN, H. *Cronobacter gen.* nov., a new genus to accommodate the biogroups of *Enterobacter sakazakii,* and proposal of *Cronobacter sakazakii* gen. nov., comb. nov. Cronobacter *malonaticus* sp. nov., Cronobacter *turicensis* sp. nov., Cronobacter *muytjensiisp. nov, Cronobacter genomospecies* 1, and of three subspecies, Cronobacter *dublinensis subsp.* Dublinensis subsp. nov., *Cronobacter dublinensis subsp.* lausannensis subsp. nov. and *Cronobacter dublinensis subsp.* Lactaridi subsp. nov. *International Journal of Systematic and Evolutionary Microbiology.* v. 58, p.1442-1447. 2008.

JENSEN, R. G. The composition of bovine milk lipids: January 1995 to December 2000. *Journal of Dairy Science,* v. 85, n. 2, p. 295-350. 2002.

JOHNSON, P. E.; EVANS, G. W. Relative zinc availability in human breast milk, infant formulas, and cow's milk. *The American Journal of Clinical Nutrition,* v. 31, p. 416-421. 1978.

KAARME, J.; HASAN, B.; RASHID, M.; OLSEN, B. Zero Prevalence of Vancomycin-Resistant Enterococci Among Swedish Preschool Children. *Microbiology Drug Resistance.* v. 0. n. 0. Feb. 2015.

KALYANTANDA, G.; SHUMYAK, L.; ARCHIBALD, L. K. *Cronobacter* species contamination of powdered infant formula and the implications for neonatal health. *Frontiers in Pediatrics.* v. 3, Jul. 2015.

KASHLAN, N. B.; HASSAN, A. S.; SRIVASTAVA, V. P.; MOHANA, N. A.; SHUBBER, K. M. Elemental contents of milk-based and soy-based infant formulas marketed in Kuwait. *Food Chemistry,* v. 42, p. 57-64. 1991.

KASNOWSKI, M. C.; MANTILLA, S. P. S.; OLIVEIRA, L. A. T.; FRANCO, R. M. Biofilm formation in the food industry and surface validation methods. *Revista científica eletrónica de medicina veterinária,* n. 15, p. 23. 2010.

KENNEDY, J.; BLAIR, I. S.; McDOWELL, D. A.; BOLTON, D. J. An investigation of the thermal inactivation of *Staphylococcus aureus* and the potential for increased thermotolerance as a result of chilled storage. *Journal of Applied Microbiology,* v. 99, p. 1229-1235. 2005.

KIM, E. K.; SHON, D. H.; RYU, D.; PARK, J. W.; HWANG, H. J.; KIM, Y. B. Occurrence of aflatoxin M1 in Korean dairy products determined by ELISA and HPLC. *Food Additives and Contaminants,* v. 17, n. 1, p. 59-64, 2000.

KIM, S.; PARK, J. Thermal Resistance and Inactivation of *Enterobacter sakazakii* Isolates during Rehydration of Powdered Infant Formula. *Journal of Microbiology and Biotechnology,* v. 17, n. 2, p. 364-368. 2007.

KLICH, M. A. *Identification of common Aspergillus species.* Netherlends. Central bureau voor Schinmelcultures, 2002. 116p.

KORNACKI, J. L.; GURTLER, J. B.; STAWICK, B. A. *Enterobacteriaceae,* Coliforms, and *Escherichia coli* as Quality and Safety indicators in *Compendium of Methods for the Microbiological Examination of Foods,* 5 ed.

LANÇAS, P. M. Modern liquid chromatography and mass spectrometry: finally "compatible"?, *Scientia Chromatographica,* São Paulo, v. 1, n. 2, p. 35-61, 2009.

LEAL, D. Growth of food outside the home. *Food Security and Nutrition,* v. 17, n. 1, p. 123-132. 2010.

LEHNER, A.; STEPHAN, R. Microbiological, epidemiological and food safety aspects of *Enterobacter sakazakii. Journal of Food Protection,* v. 67, n. 12, p. 2850-2857. 2004.

LOGAN, N. A.; VOS, P. D. *Bacillus.in Bergey's Manual of Systematics of Archaea and Bacteria.* 2015.

LONNERDALL, B. Regulation of mineral and trace elements in human milk exogenous and endogenous factors. *Nutrition Reviews*, v. 58, n.8, p. 223-229. 2000.

LOPEZ, M. I.; PETTIS, J. S.; SMITH, I. B.; CHU, P. Multiclass determination and confirmation of antibiotic residues in honey using LC-MS/MS. *Journal of Agricultural and Food Chemistry*, v. 56, p. 1553-1559, 2008.

MAHAN, L.K.; ESCOTT-STUMP, S. *Alimentos, nutrição e dietoterapia.* 9ª ed. São Paulo: ROCA. 1998.

MARRONI, I. V.; ZANATTA, Z. G. C. N.; CASAGRANDE JUNIOR, J. G.; UENO, B.; MOURA, A. B. Efeito do tratamento com calor seco e água quente sobre a germinação e controle de micro-organismos associados às sementes de mamoneira. *Arquivos do Instituto Biológico,* v. 76, n. 4, p. 761-767. 2009.

MARTINS-DINIZ, J. N.; SILVA, R. A. M.; MIRANDA, E. T.; MENDES-GIANNINNI, M. J. S. Monitoramento de fungos anemófilos e de leveduras em unidade hospitalar. *Revista Saúde Pública,* v. 39, n. 3, p. 398-405. 2005.

MERCK, *Microbiology Manual,* Berlin. Germany, 2002. 407 p.

MERCK, 2002, modified by: FRANCO, R. M.; MANTILLA, S. P. S. *Escherichia coli* in beef cuts (chuck): evaluation of methodology and antimicrobial sensitivity to predominant serovars. In: SEMINÁRIO DE INICIAÇÃO CIENTÍFICA E PRÊMIO UFF VASCONCELOS TORRES DE CIÊNCIA E TECNOLOGIA, 14, 2004, Rio de Janeiro. **Annals...**Rio de Janeiro: UFF, 2004. CD. For use in CD.

MEUCCI, V.; RAZZUOLI, E.; SOLDANI, G.; MASSART, P. Mycotoxin detection in infant formula milks in Italy. *Food Additives & Contaminants:* Part A, v. 27, n. 1, p. 6471. 2010.

MITCHELL, J. M.; GRIFFITHS, M. W.; McEWEN, S. A.; McNAB, W. B. YEE, A. J. Antimicrobial Drug Residues in Milk and Meat: Causes, Concerns, Prevalence, Regulations, Tests, and Test Performance. *Journal of Food Protection,* v. 61, v.6, p. 742-756. 1998.

MOBIN, M.; SALMITO, M. A. Microbiota fúngica dos condicionadores de air nas unidades de terapia intensiva de Teresina, PI. *Revista da Sociedade Brasileira de Medicina Tropical,* v. 36, n. 6, p. 556-559. 2006.

MONTANARI, C.; SERRAZANETTI, D. I.; FELIS, G.; TORRIANI, S.; TABANELLI, G. LANCIOTTI, R.; GARDINI, P. New insights in thermal resistance of staphylococcal strains belonging to the species *Staphylococcus epidermidis, Staphylococcus lugdunensis* and *Staphylococcus aureus. Food Control,* v. 50, p. 605-612. 2015.

MOURA, P. L. C.; MAIHARA, V. A.; CASTRO, L. P.; FIGUEIRA, R. C. L. Essential trace elements in edible mushrooms by Neutron Activation Analysis. In: *International Nuclear Atlantic Conference INAC 2007* (VIII ENAN), 2007, Santos. Proceedings of the International Nuclear Atlantic Conference 2007- INAC 2007 (VIII ENAN), v. 1, p. 1 6. 2007.

MOURA, A. C.; TASCA, A. C.; PINTO, P. G. da S.; SOARES, A.; ASSUMPÇÃO, R. B. Microbiological quality of wheat flour (Triticum aestivum) commercialized in the city of

Cascavel (Paraná). *Segurança Alimentar e Nutricional,* v. 21, n. 2, p. 499504. 2014.

NASCIMENTO, G. G. P.; MAESTRO, V.; CAMPOS, M. S. P. Ocorrência de residuos de antibióticos no leite comercializado em Piracicaba, SP. *Revista de Nutrição,* v.14, n.2, p. 119-124. 2001.

NELSON, P. T.; TOUSSOIN, T. A. A; MARASAS, W. E. O. (Eds.) *Fusarium* species. An illustrated manual for identification. The Pennsylvania State University Press, University Park, PA, London. 1983.

NEMA, V.; AGRAWAL, R.; KAMBOJ, D. V.; GOEL, A. K.; SINGH, L. Isolation and characterization of heat resistant enterotoxigenic *Staphylococcus aureus* from a food poisoning outbreak in Indian subcontinent. *International Journal of Food Microbiology,* v. 117, p. 29-35. 2007.

NES, I. P., DIEP, D. B., IKE, Y. Enterococcal Bacteriocins and Antimicrobial Proteins that Contribute to Niche Control. In: GILMORE M. S.; CLEWELL D. B.; IKE Y.; SHANKAR N. editors. *SourceEnterococci: From Commensals to Leading Causes of Drug Resistant Infection.* Boston: Massachusetts. Massachusetts Eye and Ear Infirmary, 2014, 674p.

NETTO, D. P.; LOPES, M. O.; OLIVEIRA, M. C. S.; NUNES, M. P.; MACHINSKI JUNIOR, M.; BOSQUIROLI, S. L.; BENATTO, A.; BENINI, A.; BOMBARDELLI, A. L.

C.; VEDOVELLO FILHO, D.; MACHADO, E.; BELMONTE, I. L.; ALBERTON, M.; PEDROSO, P. P.; SCUCATO, E. S. Survey of the main drugs used in dairy cattle in the State of Paraná. *Acta Scientiarum. Animal Science,* v. 27, n. 1, p. 145-151.2005.

NIENOV, A. T.; MACEDO, M. B.; FÉLIX, C.; RAMOS, D.; MOREIRA, Â. N.; SILVA, P. E. A. Hygienic-sanitary quality of infant formulas given to neonates. *Nutrire: revista da Sociedade Brasileira de Alimentação e nutrição,* v. 34, n. 2, p. 127-138. 2009.

NJONGMENTA, N. A.; HALL, P. A.; LEDENBACH, L.; FLOWERS, R. S. Acid Producing Microorganisms in *Compendium of Methods for the Microbiological Examination of Foods,* 5 ed.

NRC. National Research Council. *An Evaluation of the Role of Microbiological Criteria for Foods and Food Ingredients.* National Academy Press, Washington D.C, 1985. OLIVEIRA, J. C. *Tópicos em Micologia Médica.* 4°ed. Rio de Janeiro. 2014. 230p.

OLIVEIRA, M. N. *Tecnologia de produtos lácteos funcionais.* São Paulo: Editora Atheneu. 2009. 384p.

OLIVEIRA, C. A. P.; GERMANO, P. M. L. Avaliação do desempenho do método do ensaio por enzimas imuno-adsorvidas (ELISA) em leite em pó reconstituído contaminado experimentalmente com aflatoxina M1. *Revista Saúde Pública,* v. 30, n. 6, p.542-548. 1996.

WHO. WORLD HEALTH ORGANIZATION. United Nations Children's Fund, Ministry of Health. *Guia de avaliação de Hospital Amigo da Criança.* Brasília: Ministry of Health; 2009.

ORDÓNEZ, J. A. *Tecnologia de Alimentos*. Porto Alegre: Artmed. 2005. 280 p.

OSAILI, T. M.; SAKER, R. R.; AL-HADDAQ, M. S.; AL-NABULSI, A. A.; HOLLEY, R. A. Heat resistance of *Cronobacterspecies (Enterobacter sakazakii)* in milk and special feeding formula. *Journal of Applied Microbiology*, v. 107, p. 928-935. 2009.

PITT, J.L.; HOCKING, A.D. *Fungi and food*. London: Black Academy & Professional Chapmam & Hall, 1998. 593p.

POPOFF, M. Y.; LE MINOR, L. E. *Salmonella*. In: Bergey's Manual of Systematics of Archaea and Bacteria. 2015.

QUADROS, M. E.; LISBOA, H. de M.; OLIVEIRA, V. L.; SCHIRMER, W. N. Air quality in hospital indoor environments: case study and critical analysis of current standards. *Revista Engenharia Sanitária*, v. 14, n. 3, p. 431-438. 2009.

RAISON-PEYRON, N.; MESSAAD, D.; BOUSQUET, J.; DEMOLY, P. Anaphylaxis to beef in penicillin-allergic patient. *Allergy*, v. 56, n. 8, p. 796-797, 2001.

REGINATO, A.; PENA, P. de L.; TRENTO, P. K. S.; GIODARNO, L. C. R. S.; KINCHOKU, H.; ANTUNES, A. E.C. Microbiological quality of infant formulas administered in a public hospital in the municipality of Campinas, São Paulo. *Segurança Alimentar e Nutricional, Campinas*. v. 21. n. 1. p. 387-394. 2014.

REIS, V. B. M. *Detecção E Caracterização Bioquímica e Molecular De Bacillus cereus Em Grains*. 2012. 78 p. Dissertation (Master in Biotechnology) - Universidade de Caxias do Sul, 2012.

REZENDE-LAGO, N. C. M.; ROSSI JR, O. D.; VIDAL-MARTINS, A. M. C.; AMARAL, L. A. Occurrence of Bacillus cereus in whole milk and enterotoxigenic capacity of isolated strains. *Arquivo Brasileiro de Medicina Veterinária e Zootecnia*, v. 59, n. 6, p. 1563-1569. 2007.

RODRIGUES, M. X.; DALL'AGNOLB, L.; BITTENCOURTA, J. V. M. Survey of the occurrence of antibiotic residues in raw milk produced in the Campos Gerais region, Paraná. *UNOPAR Científica Ciência Biologicas e Saúde*, n. 14, v. 4, p. 237240, 2012.

ROSSI P.; KABUKI D. Y.; KUAYE A. Y. Avaliação microbiológica do preparo de fórmula láctea infantil em lactário hospitalar. *Revista do Instituto Adolfo Lutz*, v. 69, n. 4, p.503-509. 2010.

RYSER, E. T.; SCHUMAN, J. D. Mesophilic Aerobic Plate Count in *Compendium of Methods for the Microbiological Examination of Foods*, 5 ed.

SALIMENA, A. P. S. Biofilm formation in the food industry by *staphylococcus aureus* strains isolated from bovine mastitis. *CES Magazine*, v. 28, n. 1, p. 88102. 2014.

SALOMÃO, B. C. M.; CHUREY, J. J.; ARAGÃO, G. M. P.; WOROBO, R. W. Modeling Penicillium expansum Resistance to Thermal and Chlorine Treatments. *Journal of Food Protection*, v. 72, n. 12, p. 2618-2622. 2009.

SAMSON, R.A.; ELLEN S.H.; FRISVARD J. *Introduction to food-and airborne fungi.*

No. Ed. 7. Centraalbureau voor Schimmelcultures (CBS), 2004, 389 p.

SANTOS, J. S.; OKANO, W.; ARRAIS, B. C. D.; COSTABEBER, I. H.; SANTANA, E. H. W. Aflatoxin M1 in Dairy Products and Acid Lactic Bacteria as Biocontrol Agent in Milk. *Uniciências,* v. 18, n. 1, p. 51-56. 2014.

SANTOS, M. I. S.; TONDO, E. C. Determinação de perigos e pontos críticos de controle para implantação de sistema de análise de perigos e pontos críticos de controle em lactário. *Revista de Nutrição,* v. 13, n. 3, p. 211-222. 2000.
São Paulo, v. 64, n. 2, p.187-191, 2002.

SCHLEIFER, K.H.; BELL, J. A. *Staphylococcus.* In: *Bergey's Manual of Systematics of Archaea and Bacteria.* 2015.

SCHOENI, J. L.; WONG, A.C.L. *Bacillus cereus* Food Poisoning and its Toxins *Journal of Food Protection,* v.68, n.3, p.636-648. 2005.

SCOTT, P.M. Natural Toxins. *In:* Cunnif, P. (ed). *Official Methods of Analysis of Association of Official Analytical Chemists.* Gaithersburg, Maryland, 1997, 970.

SHAO, S.; JIA, X.; ZHANG, J.; MENG, J.; WU, H.; DUAN, H.; TU, X. Multi-residual analysis of 16 beta-agonists in pig liver, kidney and muscle by ultra performance liquid chromatography tandem mass spectrometry. *Food Chemistry,* v. 114, n. 3, p. 11151121, 2009.

SHEARER, A. E. H.; MAZZOTTA, A. S.; CHUYATE, R.; GOMBAS, D. E. Heat resistance of juice spoilage microorganisms. *Journal of Food Protection,* v. 65, n. 8, p. 1271-1275. 2002.

SHUNDO, L.; SABINO, M. Aflatoxin m1 in milk by immunoaffinity column cleanup with TLC/HPLC determination. *Brazilian Journal of Microbiology,v:* 37, p.164-167,2006.

SILVA, C. J.; TEJADA, T. S.; TIMM, C. D. Resistance of Salmonella isolated from humans and chickens to antimicrobials. *Revista Brasileira de Higiene e Sanidade Animal,* v. 8, n. 4, p. 120-131, 2014.

SILVA, J. M. B.; HOLLENBACH, C. B.; Fluoroquinolones X bacterial resistance in veterinary medicine. *Arquivos do Instituto Biológico,* v. 77, n. 2, p. 363-369, 2010.

SILVA, N.; JUNQUEIRA, V.C.A.; SILVEIRA, N.P.A. *Manual de métodos de Análise Microbiológica de Alimentos.* São Paulo, 1997, p.53-58.

SILVA, R. C.; ESCOBEDO, J. P.; GIOIELLI, L. A. Composição centesimal do leite humano e caracterização das propriedades físico-químicas de sua gordura. *Química Nova,* v. 30, n. 7, p. 1535-1538. 2007.

SISMOTTO, M.; PASCHOAL, J. A. R.; REYES, P. G. R. Analytical and regulatory aspects in the determination of macrolide residues in foods of animal origin by liquid chromatography associated with mass spectrometry. *Química Nova,* v.36, n.3, p.449-461, 2013.

SOARES-SANTOS, V.; BARRETO, A.; SEMEDO-LEMSADDEK, T. Characterization of Enterococci from Food and Food-Related Settings. *Journal of Food Protection.* v. 78, n. 7, p.1320-1326. 2015.

STEWART, C. M. Staphylococcus *aureus* and staphylococcal enterotoxins. In: HOCKING, A. D. (ed) *Foodborne microorganisms of public health significance.* 6 ed, Australian Institute of Food Science and Technology, Sydney. 2003. p. 359-380.

SVEC, P.; DEVRIESE, L. A. *Enterococcus.* In: Bergey's Manual of Systematics of Archaea and Bacteria. 2015.

TONHI, E.; COLLINS, K. E.; JARDIM, I. C. S. P.; COLLINS, C. H. Stationary phases for reverse phase high performance liquid chromatography (HPLC-FR) based on surfaces of functionalized inorganic oxides. *Química nova,* Campinas, v. 25, n. 4, p.616-623, 2002.

TONON, K. M.; SAVI, G. D.; SCUSSEL, V. M. Application of a LC-MS/MS method for multimycotoxin analysis in infant formula and milkbased products for young children commercialized in Southern Brazil. *Journal of Environmental Science and Health,* Part B, v. 0, n. 0, p. 1-7. 2018.

TRABULSI, L. B.; ALTERTHUM, P. *Microbiologia.* 5ª ed. Rio de Janeiro: Atheneu 2008. 780 p.

TROMBETE, P. M.; SANTOS, R. R.; SOUZA, A. L. R. Antibiotic residues in Brazilian milk: a review of studies published in recent years. *Revista Chilena de Nutrición,* v. 41, n. 2, p. 191-195, 2014.

TRUCKSESS, M. W. *Rapid analysis (thin layer chromatographic and immunochemical methods) for mycotoxins in foods and feeds. In:* de Koe, W.J.; Samsom, R.A.; van Egmond, H.P.; Gilbert, J.; Sabino, M. (eds). Ponsen&Looyen, Wageningen, The Netherlands, 2001, p.29-40.

USP. United State Pharmacopeia. Microbiological attributes of nonsterile nutritional and dietary supplements - *Nutritional and Dietary Supplements* <2022>. 2013.

VICTORIA, C. G.; SMITH, P. G.; VAUGHAN, J. P.; NOBRE, L. C.; LOMBARDI, C.; TEIXEIRA, A. M.; et al. Evidence for protection by breast-feeding against infant deaths from infectious diseases in Brazil. *Lancet,* 2, p. 319-22, 1987.

VIEIRA, A. A.; MOREIRA, M. E. L.; ROCHA, A. D.; PIMENTA, H. P.; LUCENA, S. L. Analysis of the energy content of human milk administered to very low birth weight newborns. *Jornal de Pediatria,* v. 80, n. 6, p.490-494. 2004.

WORLD HEALTH ORGANIZATION & FOOD AND AGRICULTURE, ORGANIZATION OF THE UNITED NATIONS. WHO. *Safety evaluation of certain mycotoxyns in food (Who Food Additivies Series 47 / FAO Food and Nutrition Paper).* Geneva, 2001.

WORLD HEALTH ORGANIZATION & FOOD AND AGRICULTURE, ORGANIZATION OF THE UNITED NATIONS. *WHODiet, nutrition, and the prevention of chronic diseases: report of a joint WHO/FAO expert consultation* (Vol. 916). Geneva, 2003.

WORLD HEALTH ORGANIZATION & UNITED NATIONS CHILDREN'S

FOUNDATION.
WHO. *Global strategy for infant and young child feeding.* Geneva, 2009

WORLD HEALTH ORGANIZATION, UNITED NATIONS CHILDREN'S FOUNDATION.
WHO. *Acceptable medical reasons for use of breast-milk substitutes.* Geneva, 2009a

WORLD HEALTH ORGANIZATION, UNITED NATIONS CHILDREN'S FOUNDATION.
WHO. *Baby-friendly hospital initiative. Revised, Updated and Expanded for Integrated Care.* Geneva, 2009b.

WORLD HEALTH ORGANIZATION, UNITED NATIONS CHILDREN'S
FUNDANTION. WHO. *Protecting, promoting and supporting breastfeeding in facilities providing maternity and newborn services: the revised Baby-friendly hospital initiative.* Geneva, 2018.

ZHENG, M. Z.; RICHARD, J. L.; BINDER, J.; A review of rapid methods for the analysis of mycotoxins. *Mycopathologia.* 161: 261-273, 2006.
*LOD: $< 1.0 \times 10^1$ CFU g^{-1} ; * **a, b and c: means with the same letter in the columns are equivalent, according to the Tukey test (P < 0.05).

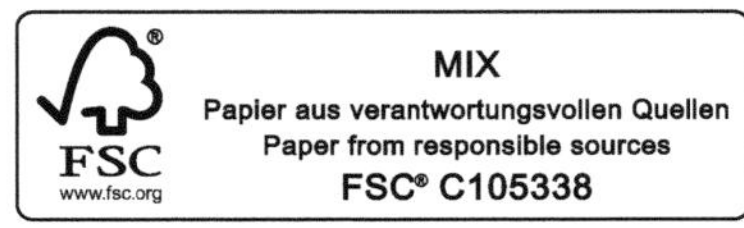

Printed by Books on Demand GmbH, Norderstedt / Germany